ADVANCES IN NEONATAL HEMATOLOGY

ADVANCES IN NEONATAL HEMATOLOGY

VIROJ WIWANITKIT

Nova Biomedical Books
New York

For permission to use material from this book please contact us:
Telephone 631-231-7269; Fax 631-231-8175
Web Site: http://www.novapublishers.com

LIBRARY OF CONGRESS CATALOGING-IN-PUBLICATION DATA

Viroj Wiwanitkit.
Advances in neonatal hematology / Viroj Wiwanitkit.
p. ; cm.
Includes bibliographical references and index.
ISBN-13: 978-1-60021-889-7 (hardcover)
ISBN-10: 1-60021-889-X (hardcover)
1. Neonatal hematology. I. Title.
[DNLM: 1. Hematologic Diseases. 2. Infant, Newborn--physiology. 3. Blood Coagulation Disorders, Inherited. WS 300 V819a 2007]
RJ269.5.V57 2007
618.92'15--dc22

2007024477

Published by Nova Science Publishers, Inc. ✦ New York

CONTENTS

Chapter 1

Physiology of Hematological System in Neonate

Neonatal red Blood Cell Physiology

Red blood cell is an important cellular component in blood stream. In neonate, red blood cells circulate in blood stream and carry oxygen to the target organ. Hemoglobin plays an important physiologic role, one that begins early in fetal development [1]. Erythropoiesis start in the utero and the complete adult system can be seen in the newborn. An important part of erythropoiesis is the hemoglobin systhesis. Basically, alpha-globin synthesis is observed in the yolk sac by 3 weeks of gestation and, by 9 weeks of gestation, alpha-globin represents the main alpha-like hemoglobin in the fetus [2]. By contrast, the switch to beta-globin chain synthesis usually remains incomplete until 1 year after birth [2]. Therefore, the clinical manifestations of homozygous beta-thalassemia may be ameliorated by sustained synthesis of fetal hemoglobin during the first 6 months of life, whereas up until 10 years ago, homozygous alpha-thalassemia was invariably associated with death in utero [2]. In the normal fetus, a switch from production of hemoglobin F (alpha 2 gamma 2) to hemoglobin A (alpha 2 beta 2) occurs at 28 to 34 weeks of gestation [3]. In the fetus with beta-hemoglobinopathy or beta-thalassemia, this switch proceeds despite the morbidity that results when production of beta-globin is abnormal or reduced [3]. The delay in the switch from gamma-globin to beta-globin under conditions of hyperinsulinemia, which occurs in infants of diabetic mothers is also noted [3]. The delay in the switch from gamma-globin to beta-globin in this unique clinical setting may allow identification of physiologic factors that can modulate developmental gene suppression [3]. Further details on the abnormality of hemoglobin synthesis can be seen in the chapters mentioning the thalassemia in this book. Another important part of hemoglobin synthesis is the heme synthesis [4]. Heme can be derived from iron. Physiologically, the majority of cells in the organism acquire iron from a well-characterized plasma glycoprotein, transferrin [4]. Iron uptake from transferrin is reasonably well understood, and involves the binding of transferrin to the transferrin receptor, internalization of transferrin within an endocytic vesicle by receptor-mediated endocytosis, and the release of iron from the protein by a decrease in endosomal pH [4]. Most of the transferrin-bound iron is used for the synthesis of hemoglobin by developing erythroid cells [4].

It can be seen that iron is a very important trace element [5-6]. Negative iron balance throughout pregnancy, particularly in the latter half, may lead to iron deficiency anaemia during the third trimester [7]. The increase in iron demand is required to meet the expansion in maternal haemoglobin mass and to meet the needs of fetal growth [7]. Fetal demand for iron results in a unidirectional flow of iron to the fetus against a concentration gradient regulated by fetal requirements for iron; this iron transfer occurs almost entirely irrespective of maternal iron status [7]. Iron deficiency during pregnancy affects a significant portion of women in countries with low economic wealth and is not uncommon in pregnant women in industrialized countries [6]. Inadequate intake of iron related to diets poor in bioavailable iron is often responsible for iron deficiency before pregnancy, and metabolic adjustments (such as mobilization of iron stores and increased absorption) are insufficient to meet increasing needs during pregnancy [6]. Off-spring of iron deficient mothers have decreased iron stores and may develop anaemia in the first year of life [5]. Studies have shown behavioural abnormalities in children with iron deficiency and poor performance in the Bayley Mental Developmental Index [5]. The presence of iron is necessary for the metabolic processes, erythropoiesis, oxygen transport and respiration, thermoregulation and humoral and cellular immunity [8]. Congenital fetal malformations and intrauterine growth retardation might be also stimulated by iron deficiency [8].Therefore, it is recommended to provide iron supplementation to the pregnant [9].

The physiology of maternal and fetal erythropoiesis in pregnancy shows that hematopoiesis, and the stimulation of hematopoiesis, take place separately in the two circulations [9]. Erythropoietin appears the main regulator in both mother and fetus [10]. The human placenta forms a manifest barrier to endogenous and recombinant erythropoietin, thus fulfilling the cardinal precondition for the use of recombinant erythropoietin in the treatment of maternal pregnancy anemia [10]. The mechanisms controlling the expression of the gene encoding for the hormone erythropoietin are exemplary for oxygen-regulated gene expression [11]. In humans and other mammals, hypoxia modulates erythropoietin levels by increasing expression of the erythropoietin gene [11]. In fetus life erythropoiesis takes place in yolk sack first, then in liver and after that in bone marrow [12]. Erythropoietin participates in liver erythropoiesis and in bone marrow [12]. Until recently, the major site of erythropoietin production in the fetus was thought to be the liver, but studies have shown now that the erythropoietin gene is expressed strongly in the fetal kidney, even in the temporary mesonephros [13]. The metanephric erythropoietin mRNA is upregulated by anemia, downregulated by glucocorticoids, and contributes substantially to circulating hormone levels in hemorrhaged ovine fetuses [13]. Other sites of erythropoietin and erythropoietin receptor production, likely to have important actions during development, are the placenta and the brain [13]. Polycythemia which appears in newborns after delivery is the result of fetus hypozemic metabolic constellation, which leads to excessive erythropoietin production [12]. The substitution of HbF biosynthesis way to HbA is supposedly the reason of erythropoietin secretion drop after delivery [12]. During first 3 months of newborn life erythropoietin secretion stimulation takes place at a lower then adults' blood hemoglobin level [12]. Nonerythropoietic roles of the erythropoietin are also mentioned [14]. Areas in which erythropoietin has important recognized effects are on endothelial cells, and in the developing heart, gastrointestinal tract, and brain [14]. It may also be important in the regulation of vascular growth during the menstrual cycle, and in the stimulation of testosterone production in men [14]. Erythropoietin is prominent in the brain during fetal development, leading to speculation that they play an important role in neurodevelopment [14]. There are also promising data regarding erythropoietin as a possible neuroprotective agent in such conditions as hypoxia, because it decreases programmed cell death induced during such adverse conditions [14]. It has been known for many decades that oxidative stress leads to oxidation of hemoglobin and damage to the erythrocyte membrane [15]. More recently, the factors involved in denaturating of membrane proteins and lipid peroxidation have been investigated in detail, as well as the mechanism of reactive oxygen species formation in red cells [15]. The recent insight into the mechanism of oxidative injury of red cells and evidence of relationships between erythrocyte oxidative stress and hypoxia suggest that increased hemolysis is induced by severe hypoxia and acidosis in the fetus as well as the newborn [15].

Plasma membrane and cell surface changes during erythroid maturation is observed [16-18]. Basically, the major integral proteins comprise the anion transport protein (band 3), the glucose transporter and four sialic acid-rich polypeptides [19]. The anion transport protein equilibrates Cl- and HCO-3 between the plasma and red cell and also provides an anchorage site for peripheral proteins including those in the red cell cytoskeleton [19]. The sialic acid-rich proteins are predominantly exposed at the surface of the cell [19]. The bulk of the peripheral proteins are organized in a complex fashion to form a skeletal meshwork at the cytoplasmic surface of the membrane which maintains the shape and deformability of the red cell [17]. Fukuda et al found that the profiles of oligosaccharides released by endo-β-galactosidase and immunofluorescence studies with anti-Ii antibodies indicated that a linear polylactosaminoglycan structure was present in erythroblasts as well as in erythrocytes of the fetal and newborn stage, whereas a branched polylactosaminoglycan structure was present in erythroblasts as well as erythrocytes of adult blood [17]. They concluded that two membrane characteristics were closely associated with the process of erythroid cell development; one, the membrane proteins band 3, band 4.5, and 95- and 105-kilodalton glycoproteins which determined the degree of maturation, and the other, polylactosaminoglycan, which might determine the ontogenic stage of the erythroblast progenitors [17]. Developmental process of red blood cell membrane plays important roles in determination of red blood cell enzyme activity. During fetal development, antioxidant defense mechanisms have generally been considered to be less active than those of mature newborn infants or of the adults [20]. It has been suggested that this might reflect a lower requirement for cellular antioxidant activity because of the relatively protective intrauterine environment and the lower perfusing oxygen tension in the fetus [20]. Erythrocyte superoxide dismutase and Cu, Zn-superoxide dismutase in plasma blood changed significantly with maturation, by term Cu, Zn-superoxide dismutase activity reached a level higher than in adults [20]. High superoxide dismutase activity, perhaps, is one of biochemical specific preparation for birth occurs in developing fetus to help assure it's successful adaptation to comparatively O2-rich world at birth [20]. Maturational changes in the activity of the red cell enzymes are apparent from about 31-36 week of gestation, suggesting that the stimulation for these changes may have commenced from about 28-31 week [21].

Neonatal white Blood Cell Physiology

White blood cell is an important cellular component in blood stream. In neonate, white blood cells circulate in blood stream and play important role in several defense mechanisms. Concerning white blood cell development, there are two main processes, myelopoiesis and lymphopoiesis. Myelopoiesis is the process of development of polymorphonuclear cell (nutrophil, eosinophil, basophile) and monocyte while lymphopoeiesis is the process of development of lymphocyte (both B and T cells). Myelopoieis starts in utero, in the same time as erythropoiesis. In fetal liver, myelopoietic cells were localized mainly around portal triad vessels and increased in number with gestational age while lymphoid precursors scatter among the hepatocytes without any sign of focal development in the age range [22]. Unlike erythropoiesis, the information on myelopoiesis and lymphopoiesis is limited. For myelopoiesis, the early stages of granulopoiesis are mediated by the C/EBPalpha, PU.1, RAR, CBF, and c-Myb transcription factors, and the later stages require C/EBPepsilon, PU.1, and CDP. Monocyte development requires PU.1 and interferon consensus sequence binding protein and can be induced by Maf-B, c-Jun, or Egr-1 [23]. Cytokine receptor signals modulate transcription factor activities but do not determine cell fates [23]. Several mechanisms orchestrate the myeloid developmental program, including cooperative gene regulation, protein:protein interactions, regulation of factor levels, and induction of cell cycle arrest [23-24]. The vitamin A derivative retinoic acid plays a critical role during the differentiation of myeloid progenitors towards the neutrophil lineage [25]. This role is primarily mediated by binding of retinoic acid to retinoic acid receptor alpha (RARalpha), a nuclear receptor that modulates the expression of multiple downstream targets via retinoic acid response elements [25]. In the newborn, the myelopoiesis is complete, the neutrophil, eosinophil, basophile and monocyte are clearly separated.

It has long been controversial whether hematopoiesis progresses through ordered stages of determination as in embryonic development. It was recently found that the process of lineage commitment proceeded through an ordered but not random process [26]. Stepwise lineage restriction of progenitors in lympho-myelopoiesis can be identified [26]. For lymphopoiesis, interleukin (IL)-7 is a growth and differentiation factor for gammadelta T cells but a growth factor only for alphabeta T cells [27]. IL-7 is constitutively expressed in the thymus, bone marrow stromal cells, epithelial and dendritic cells, keratinocytes, as well as in fetal and adult liver [28]. IL-7 acts on various cells through its receptor (IL-7R), a heterodimer consisting of an alpha chain (CD127) that specifically binds IL-7 and a common gamma(c) chain (CD132) shared by other cytokine receptors [28]. The receptor is expressed on bone marrow progenitor cells, lymphoid T and B precursors, and mature T cells [28]. T-cell development in the thymus requires periodic importation of hematopoietic progenitors from the bone marrow [29-30]. Such thymus settling progenitors arise from hematopoietic stem cells that are retained in a specific bone marrow microenvironmental niche [29-30]. Thymic lymphopoiesis depends on blood-borne, marrow-derived progenitors, but characterization of these cells, and their lineage potentials, has been difficult [29]. The full development of intrathymic hematopoiesis depends upon the successful completion of a series of well coordinated cellular interactions between widely divergent cells such as epithelium (primitive pharynx); ectomesenchyrne (neural crest); and PHSCs (yolk sac, fetal liver) [31]. The human thymus is a generalized hematopoietic tissue with between 7 to 9 week of ontogenesis [31]. In human fetuses various elements of mammalian hematopoiesis were identified intrathymically: B lymphocytes, plasma cells, erythropoietic and granulocytopoietic (neutrophils and eosinophils) cells, antigen presenting dendritic cells, and mast cells [31]. In addition to thymus, the lymph nodes harbor a cryptic T-lymphopoietic pathway that is dramatically amplified by oncostatin M [32]. Extrathymic T cells undergo enhanced homeostatic proliferation and thereby acquire some properties of memory T cells [32]. Following antigen encounter, extrathymic T-cells initiate proliferation and cytokine secretion more readily than classic T cells, but their accumulation is limited by an exquisite susceptibility to apoptosis [32].

For B cell, most are produced in the bone marrow. Transcription factors including PU.1, E2A and early B cell factor (EBF) are essential for the earliest stages of B lymphocyte development [33]. Recent advances suggest that, although PU.1 initiates events leading to B lymphopoiesis, it might be dispensable at later stages of development [33]. B cell development is also a process tightly regulated by the orchestrated signaling of cytokine receptors, the pre-B cell receptor and the B cell receptor [34]. It commences with common lymphoid progenitors up-regulating the expression of B cell-related genes and committing to the B cell lineage [35]. The production of B lymphocytes begins to decline steadily early in adult life and is severely compromised in the elderly [35].

NEONATAL PLATELET PHYSIOLOGY

Platelet is a part of blood cell in the blood circulation. Megakaryocyte is the marrow cell that gives rise to platelet. It has important role in hemostasis. The knowledge on the platelet is fewer than those of red blood cell and white blood cell. C-mpl ligand or thrombopoietin (Tpo) is increasingly recognised as the major regulator of platelet homeostasis in humans [36]. Preliminary studies in neonates showing increased Tpo levels most often during thrombocytopenia accompanied by reduced megakaryocytopoiesis supports this concept [36]. In addition to this demonstrable fetal and neonatal endogenous Tpo production megakaryocyte progenitor and precursor cells from the fetus and from preterm and term newborns proliferate and differentiate extensively in-vitro in response to exogenous Tpo [36]. Murray et al strongly suggested that strongly suggest that: 1) Tpo is a major regulator of megakaryocytopoiesis/platelet production in the fetus/newborn, 2) impaired fetal Tpo production may be a factor in early thrombocytopenia in preterm babies, and 3) recombinant human Tpo is likely to be effective in the treatment of early neonatal thrombocytopenia [37]. In thrombopoiesis, Tpo affects nearly all aspects of platelet production, from self-renewal and expansion of HSCs, through stimulation of the proliferation of megakaryocyte progenitor cells, to support of the maturation of these cells into platelet-producing cells [38]. How a megakaryocyte originates from a hematopoietic stem cell and how this cell undergoes further maturation and differentiation is a complex process, controlled at different stages by several transcription factor [39]. These transcription factors influence the expression of their own target genes, leading to megakaryocyte maturation and platelet release [39]. One of the transcription factors that is most studied in this regard is GATA1, that forms a transcriptional complex with its cofactor FOG1 [39]. The process of megakaryopoiesis occurs in utero in the same phase as erythropoiesis and myelopoiesis. For laboratory investigation, high levels of reticulated platelets and thrombopoietin can effectively characterize fetal thrombopoiesis [40]. For the newborn, thrombocytopoiesis is more active in female than in male [41]. In comparison with adults or children, the hemostasis of newborn infants, although physiological, is characterized by a reduced functional reserve capacity leading to the rapid occurrence of bleeding disorders especially in the presence of additional risk factors such as prematurity, asphyxia, or infection [42]. Morphological and biochemical differences reflect an immature cellular stage which results in platelet hyporeactivity and contributes to the reduced capacity of the neonatal haemostatic system [42].

NEONATAL HEMOSTASIS PHYSIOLOGY

Generally, hemostasis consists of two important parts, coagulation and fibrinolysis. Considering coagulation system, placental trophoblasts express and produce coagulation components, participating not only in hemostasis but also in placental vascular development and differentiation [43]. The expression of tissue factor, membrane phosphatidylserine and fibrin render the trophoblasts pro-coagulant, thus compromising the risk of bleeding while exposing the placenta to pro-thrombotic risks [43]. Local inhibitory mechanisms-TFPI-1 and TFPI-2, thrombomodulin, annexin V and the fibrinolytic system-limit coagulation activation and fibrin deposition [43]. In newborn, the coagulation system is complete and has full function to response to bleeding episode. The success of coagulation system consists of coagulation factor, vascular component as well as platelet. More information on the bleeding disorder in the neonate can be seen in another chapter in this book. However, newborn infants are at risk for developing haemorrhage or thrombosis when provoked by various pathological stimuli [44]. Hemostasis screening tests and factor assays must be interpreted using gestational age-specific normal ranges [44]. In human, the fibrinolytic system comprises a series of serine proteases that interact to cleave fibrin into fibrin degradation products [45]. Although all key components of the fibrinolytic system are present at birth, important age-dependent, quantitative and qualitative differences are present during childhood as compared to adults [45]. These differences include decreased plasma concentrations of plasminogen, tissue-type plasminogen activator and alpha2-antiplasmin, increased plasma concentrations of plasminogen activator inhibitor-1, as well as a decrease in both plasmin generation and overall fibrinolytic activity [45]. Although all components of the fibrinolytic system are present at birth, plasma concentrations of key components in infants and children differ physiologically from those in adults [46]. Until the age of 6 months, plasma concentrations of plasminogen and alpha (2)-antiplasmin are decreased to 50% and 80% of adult values, respectively, while plasma concentrations of tissue-type plasminogen activator are decreased and plasminogen activator inhibitor-1 are increased throughout childhood [46].

Blood Collection in Neonate

Blood collection is important medical procedure. It is useful for getting blood sample for laboratory analysis. Basically, the amount of collected blood is very few comparing to the human body. However, it can be considered important in the neonate. In neonate, blood collection should be carefully done and should be performed only if necessary. Routinely, venepucture is the a common blood collection procedure. Both syringe and evacuated systems can be applied. But the syringe blood collection is more preferable than evacuated blood collection in the neonatal. The site of venipuncture is sometimes different from the adult. The common site is the scalp vein with usage of butterfly set. It should be noted that capillary blood collection should be replaced venipuncture if it is allowable. The amount of collected blood is usually little. Sometimes, 1 drops smeared on the filter paper is acceptable for further laboratory analysis.

References

[1] Bell SG. An introduction to hemoglobin physiology. *Neonatal Netw.* 1999 Mar;18(2):9-15.

[2] Olivieri NF. Fetal erythropoiesis and the diagnosis and treatment of hemoglobin disorders in the fetus and child. *Semin Perinatol.* 1997 Feb;21(1):63-9.

[3] Perrine SP, Greene MF, Faller DV. Delay in the fetal globin switch in infants of diabetic mothers. *N Engl J Med.* 1985 Feb 7;312(6):334-8.

[4] Ponka P, Beaumont C, Richardson DR. Function and regulation of transferrin and ferritin. *Semin Hematol.* 1998 Jan;35(1):35-54.

[5] Letsky EA. Erythropoiesis in pregnancy. *J Perinat Med.* 1995; 23(1-2):39-45.

[6] Blot I, Diallo D, Tchernia G. Iron deficiency in pregnancy: effects on the newborn. *Curr Opin Hematol.* 1999 Mar;6(2):65-70.

[7] Bentley DP. Iron metabolism and anaemia in pregnancy. *Clin Haematol.* 1985 Oct;14(3):613-28.

[8] Zdziennicki A, Laudanski T. Iron deficiency as a risk factor during the perinatal period. *Ginekol Pol.* 1996 Jun;67(6):301-3.

[9] Haider BA, Bhutta ZA. Multiple-micronutrient supplementation for women during pregnancy. *Cochrane Database Syst Rev.* 2006 Oct 18;(4):CD004905.

[10] Huch R, Huch A. Erythropoietin in obstetrics. *Hematol Oncol Clin North Am.* 1994 Oct;8(5):1021-40.

[11] Stockmann C, Fandrey J. Hypoxia-induced erythropoietin production: a paradigm for oxygen-regulated gene expression. *Clin Exp Pharmacol Physiol.* 2006 Oct;33(10):968-79.

[12] Ulman I. The role of erythropoietin in erythropoiesis regulation in fetuses and newborn infants. *Ginekol Pol.* 1996 Apr;67(4):205-9.

[13] Moritz KM, Lim GB, Wintour EM. Developmental regulation of erythropoietin and erythropoiesis. *Am J Physiol.* 1997 Dec;273(6 Pt 2):R1829-44.

[14] Juul SE. Nonerythropoietic roles of erythropoietin in the fetus and neonate. *Clin Perinatol.* 2000 Sep;27(3):527-41.

[15] Bracci R, Perrone S, Buonocore G. Oxidant injury in neonatal erythrocytes during the perinatal period. *Acta Paediatr Suppl.* 2002; 91(438):130-4.

[16] Fukuda M, Fukuda MN. Changes in cell surface glycoproteins and carbohydrate structures during the development and differentiation of human erythroid cells. *J Supramol Struct Cell Biochem.* 1981;17(4):313-24.

[17] Fukuda M, Fukuda MN, Papayannopoulou T, Hakomori S. Membrane differentiation in human erythroid cells: unique profiles of cell surface glycoproteins expressed in erythroblasts in vitro from three ontogenic stages. *Proc Natl Acad Sci U S A.* 1980 Jun;77(6):3474-8.

[18] Chan LN. Plasma membrane and cell surface changes during erythroid maturation. *Prog Clin Biol Res.* 1985;184:341-53

[19] Tanner MJ. Erythrocyte membrane structure and function. *Ciba Found Symp.* 1983; 94:3-23.

[20] Krolak B, Kaminski K. Activity of superoxide dismutase (SOD) and its isoenzyme activities in newborn children and adult women and men. *Ginekol Pol.* 1992 Aug;63(8):404-9.

[21] Ripalda MJ, Rudolph N, Wong SL. Developmental patterns of antioxidant defense mechanisms in human erythrocytes. *Pediatr Res.* 1989 Oct;26(4):366-9.

[22] Timens W, Kamps WA. Hemopoiesis in human fetal and embryonic liver. *Microsc Res Tech.* 1997 Dec 1;39(5):387-97.

[23] Friedman AD. Transcriptional regulation of myelopoiesis. *Int J Hematol.* 2002 Jun;75(5):466-72.

[24] Friedman AD. Transcriptional regulation of granulocyte and monocyte development. *Oncogene.* 2002 May 13;21(21):3377-90.

[25] Gaines P, Berliner N. Retinoids in myelopoiesis. *J Biol Regul Homeost Agents.* 2003 Jan-Mar;17(1):46-65.

[26] Katsura Y, Kawamoto H. Stepwise lineage restriction of progenitors in lympho-myelopoiesis. *Int Rev Immunol.* 2001 Feb;20(1):1-20.

[27] Appasamy PM. Biological and clinical implications of interleukin-7 and lymphopoiesis. *Cytokines Cell Mol Ther.* 1999 Mar;5(1):25-39.

[28] Krawczenko A, Kieda C, Dus D. The biological role and potential therapeutic application of interleukin 7. *Arch Immunol Ther Exp (Warsz).* 2005 Nov-Dec;53(6):518-25.

[29] Petrie HT. Early commitment: T cell progenitors in the blood. *Immunity.* 2007 Jan;26(1):7-8.

[30] Schwarz BA, Bhandoola A. Trafficking from the bone marrow to the thymus: a prerequisite for thymopoiesis. *Immunol Rev.* 2006 Feb;209:47-57.

[31] Bodey B, Bodey B Jr, Siegel SE, Kaiser HE. Intrathymic non-lymphatic hematopoiesis during mammalian ontogenesis. *In Vivo.* 1998 Nov-Dec;12(6):599-618.

[32] Blais ME, Louis I, Perreault C. T-cell development: an extrathymic perspective. *Immunol Rev.* 2006 Feb;209:103-14.

[33] Hagman J, Lukin K. Transcription factors drive B cell development. *Curr Opin Immunol.* 2006 Apr;18(2):127-34

[34] Clark MR, Cooper AB, Wang LD, Aifantis I. The pre-B cell receptor in B cell development: recent advances, persistent questions and conserved mechanisms. *Curr Top Microbiol Immunol.* 2005; 290:87-103.

[35] Signer RA, Montecino-Rodriguez E, Dorshkind K. Aging, B lymphopoiesis, and patterns of leukemogenesis. *Exp Gerontol.* 2006 Dec 19.

[36] Murray NA, Watts TL, Roberts IA. Thrombopoietin in the fetus and neonate. *Early Hum Dev.* 2000 Jul;59(1):1-12.

[37] Murray NA, Watts TL, Roberts IA. Endogenous thrombopoietin levels and effect of recombinant human thrombopoietin on megakaryocyte precursors in term and preterm babies. *Pediatr Res.* 1998 Jan;43(1):148-51.

[38] Kaushansky K. The molecular mechanisms that control thrombopoiesis. *J Clin Invest.* 2005 Dec;115(12):3339-47.

[39] van Geet C. Thrombopoiesis: new concepts. *Verh K Acad Geneeskd Belg.* 2004; 66(1):5-24

[40] Jilma-Stohlawetz P, Homoncik M, Jilma B, Folman CC, von dem Borne AE, Bernaschek G, Deutinger J, Ulm B, Eppel W, Panzer S. High levels of reticulated platelets and thrombopoietin characterize fetal thrombopoiesis. *Br J Haematol.* 2001 Feb;112(2):466-8.

[41] Wasiluk A. Thrombocytopoiesis in healthy term newborns. *J Perinat Med.* 2005; 33(3):252-4.

[42] Kuhne T, Imbach P. Neonatal platelet physiology and pathophysiology. *Eur J Pediatr.* 1998 Feb;157(2):87-94.

[43] Lanir N, Aharon A, Brenner B. Haemostatic mechanisms in human placenta. *Best Pract Res Clin Haematol.* 2003 Jun;16(2):183-95.

[44] Montgomery RR, Marlar RA, Gill JC. Newborn haemostasis. *Clin Haematol.* 1985 Jun;14(2):443-60.

[45] Parmar N, Albisetti M, Berry LR, Chan AK. The fibrinolytic system in newborns and children. *Clin Lab.* 2006; 52(3-4):115-24.

[46] Albisetti M. The fibrinolytic system in children. *Semin Thromb Hemost.* 2003 Aug;29(4):339-48.

Chapter 2

NEONATAL JAUNDICE

INTRODUCTION TO BILIRUBIN

Bilirubin is the end product of red blood cell destruction process. Bilirubin is a bile pigment which results from the degradation of heme, one of the breakdown products of red blood cells [1]. It is thought to be a toxin because it is associated with neonatal jaundice, possibly leading to irreversible brain damage [1]. Formation of bilirubin is a complex biological process that consists of many steps (Figure 1).

A.hemoglobin → heme → biliverdin → insoluble bilirubin →

B. bilirubin-albumin conjugation →

C. bilirubin → bilirubin diclucoronide →

D. excreted bilirubin

Figure 1. Overview of the bilirubin production process. A is in the spleen, B is in the blood circulation, C is in the liver and D is in the intestine.

First, the aged red blood cell is entrapped into the spleen. Then the extravascular hemolysis from the reticuloendothelial system function will occur and heme is derived. The insoluble bilirubin is generated within the spleen. There are two additional important processes: 1) protein or albumin conjugation for transferring via blood circulation to liver and 2) hepatic conjugation to form the conjugated bilirubin for further excretion. The excretion of conjugated bilirubin is via the hepatobiliary system in the form of bile. Gall bladder is the reservoir of the bile. The bile will be excreted according to the stimulation of meal. Conjugated bilirubin in blie is excreted into the small intestine then pass into the large intestine. Finally, conjugated bilirubin is excreted along with feces via anus.

NEONATAL HYPERBILIRUBINEMIA

Increases bilirubin in blood is important clinical problem. The term hyperbilirubinemia is used for describing of this condition. In neonate, the hyperbilirubin is very important medical problem. The definition of neonatal hyperbilirubinemia is the condition that total serum bilirubin exceeds 5 mg/dL. It presents in up to 60 % of term newborns. This is mostly physiological, but a small percentage of these babies have pathological jaundice, requiring detailed investigations and management. here are many pathological conditions that can cause neonatal hyperbilirubinemia. Summary of important steps that pathological conditions can occur and bring neonatal hyperbilirubinemia can be seen in Figure 2. Severe complications due to neonatal hyperbilirubinemia are possible.

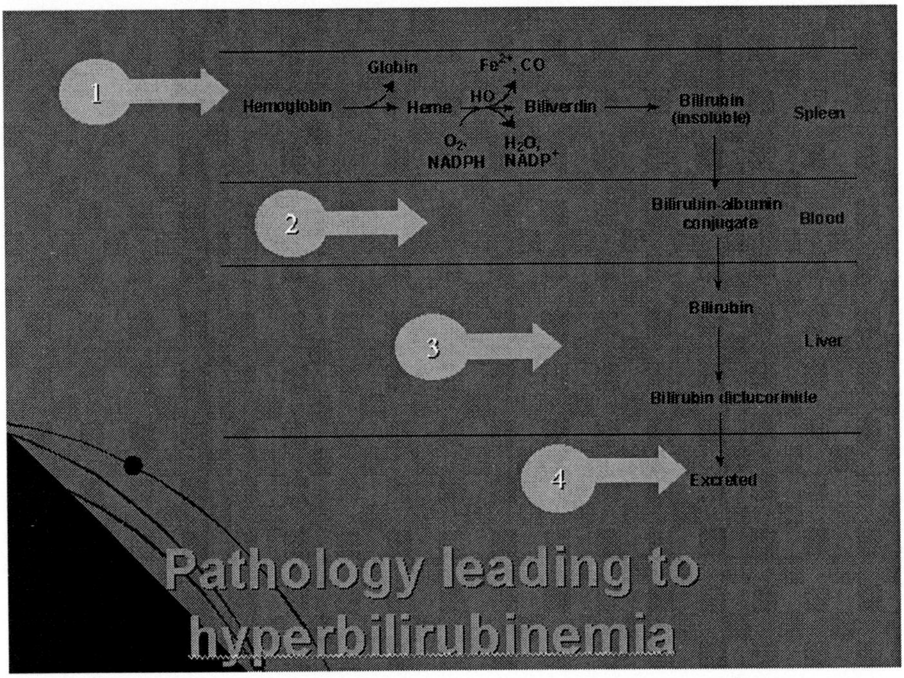

Figure 2. Summary of important steps that pathological conditions can occur and bring neonatal hyperbilirubinemia. 1 = increased bilirubin load = hemolysis; 2 = decreased albumin binding; 3 = decreased conjugation; 4 = delayed excretion = increased enterohepatic circulation.

There are four important groups of pathological conditions that can bring neonatal hyperbilirubinemia. These conditions are:

1. Increased bilirubin load or hemolysis

Increased bilirubin load due to hemolysis is an important cause of neonatal hyperbilirubinemia. Indeed, hemolysis is an important hematological disorder. There are many conditions that can cause hemolysis. The main groups are intravascular hemolysis and extravascular hemolysis [2]. The hemolysis usually coexits with anemia. Hemolytic anemia is the term for the coexistence between hemolysis and anemia [3]. In addition, the hemolytic anemia also relates with hyperbilirubinemia [4]. The common conditions that can lead hemolytic anemia in neonate include hemoglobin disorder, hemolytic disease of the newborn and red blood cell enzyme deficiency. More details on neonatal hemolysis can be seen in another chapter in this book.

2. Decreased albumin binding

Decreased albumin binding is another cause of neonatal anemia. It is usually due to the depletion of albumin in blood stream. This condition is called hypoalbuminemia. A condition that can bring hypoalbuminemia is protein malnutrition. Bilirubin-albumin binding weakens the correlation between the plasma total bilirubin concentration and bilirubin encephalopathy (kernicterus), which has led to considerable interest over the years in measuring binding as part of the evaluation of jaundiced newborns [5]. Despite development of several bilirubin-albumin binding tests, technical, ethical, and logistical factors have prevented the prospective studies needed to validate their routine clinical use [5]. The non-protein nutrition deficiency does not significantly affect the bilirubin metabolism. Another problem that can cause decreased albumin binding is the effect of drug. Some drugs can competitive bind to the albumin and cause a condition which is similar to hypoalbuminemia [6]. It should be noted that the tendency for bilirubin precipitation depends upon the ratio of unconjugated plasma bilirubin concentration to the concentration of reserve albumin for binding of bilirubin and is increased when part of the albumin is occupied by competitive binding of a drug [7].

3. Decreased conjugation

Hepatic conjugation disorder is another important cause of hyperbilirubinemia. There are several conditions that hepatic conjugation decreases. Both acquired and congenital disorders are mentioned. The important congenital disorder is Crigler-Najjar syndrome.

Crigler-Najjar syndrome is the major morbidity of this rare autosomal recessive disorder of bilirubin conjugation that results in chronic unconjugated hyperbilirubinemia [8]. Definitive prevention of the neurologic sequelae that often occur within the context of Crigler-Najjar syndrome requires that curative treatment (hepatic transplantation, presently, and gene therapy in the future) be applied prior to the possible onset of neurologic symptoms in adolescence [8]. There is another mild syndrome called Gilbert's syndrome. This syndrome is usually mild and asymptomatic. It is usually detected by accident [9]. These two syndromes are called hereditary unconjugated hyperbilirubinemias (HUHB). There is considerable evidence suggesting that genetic damages to human uridine diphosphate glucuronyltransferase (UDPGT) gene located on clhromosome 2q37 are responsible for HUHB [10]. The Crigler-Najjar syndrome of types I and II is characterized by structural mutations on one of 5 exons of HUHB gene, resulting in the synthesis of defective catalytically inactive isoforms of the enzyme [10]. In Gilbert's syndrome, genetic alterations are located at the promoter of the gene and accompanied by the nucleotide insert of thymine adenine (TA) [10]. Promoter prolongation impairs the binding of IID transcription factor and leads to the decreased production of the enzyme UDPGT 1,1 [10]. The laboratory examination by molecular diagnosis is the new advanced tool for diagnosis of neonatal hyperbilirubinemia [11].

4. Delayed excretion

Delayed excretion is another important group of condition that can cause hyperbilirubinemia. Unlike the previous three groups, the conditions in this group bring conjugated hyperbilirubinemia. The conditions are usually the obstruction of the biliary tract. Due to the obstructive mechanism, the liver function test can also revealed increased level of another important biochemical marker, alkaline phosphatase (ALP). Indeed, the biliary obstruction is one of the leading causes for both hyperalkaline phosphatasemia and hyperbilirubinemia in the neonates [12]. For the neonatal, the important condition is the biliary atresia. It is also absolutely essential to consider a possibility of extra-hepatic biliary atresia early, during management of a case of neonatal direct hyperbilirubinemia as early surgical intervention results in a better outcome [13].

Advanced Nanomolecular Pathogenesis of Neonatal Hyperbilirubinemia and its Complications

A. Energy Change in Formation of Conjugated Bilirubin [14]

Concerning the formation of conjugation, a molecule of bilirubin reacts with two molecules of glucoronic acid. The reaction occurs between OH group of proprionic acid part of bilirubin and CH group of each glucoronic acid and results in conjugated biliruin. This process is energy-dependent and occurs against a concentration gradient [15]. Physiologically, conjugation give an amount of energy to the external environment, the hepatic cell. In physiological conditation, the energy might be suitable for the hepatic environment but it might be increased in the pathological condition. Indeed, impaired or defective excretion of bilirubin, reduced glutathione and other organic anions from hepatocytes can be seen in conjugated hyperbilirubinuria rat model [16]. Granato et al found that the antiapoptotic effect of bilirubin associated with its antioxidant properties indicates that hyperbilirubinaemia may have a protective role in liver disease [17]. The nature of energy production reaction can be a good explanation. The increased giving out energy in the conjugated hyperbilirubinemia in liver disease can be a responsive mechanism to the hepatic damage in liver pathology.

The nature of energy consuming reaction in formation of conjugated bilirubin has never been reported and this can be important data for further implication in the hyperbilirubinemia. Although the bilirubin is a widely used test in clinical pathology, the exact knowledge on the energy change in the physiological conjugation of bilirubin has never been clarified. The conjugation reaction in formation of bilirubin is a type of covalent bond formation. In a recent work by Wiwanitkit [14], the required energy for conjugated bilirubin formation per molecule was calculated. Wiwanitkit found that the reaction is a type of "energy producing reaction". This finding implies several in clinical medicine.

B. Nanomolecular Pathogenesis of Kernicterus

Neonatal jaundice is an important problem in medicine [18–19]. Around 80 per cent of preterm infants develop hyperbilirubinaemia characterised by jaundice [20]. This condition is most commonly treated with phototherapy and/or exchange transfusion [20]. One of the most fatal unwanted of neonatal jaundice is kernicterus [18–19]. Historically, the presence of yellow staining and damage to the brain caused by unconjugated bilirubin was first described by Hervieux in 1847 [21]. Kernicterus, the technical term used to describe the intense yellow staining in the basal ganglia of the brain, was first used by Schmorl in 1903 [21]. Kernicterus is a preventable brain injury caused by severe jaundice, yet it remains a threat today [21]. Recent progress in understanding bilirubin binding and neurotoxicity resulting from unbound or "free" unconjugated bilirubin, how bilirubin affects the central nervous system in vivo and in vitro, and the use of new clinical tools in neonates, for example magnetic resonance imaging revealing bilateral lesions in globus pallidus and subthalamus, and abnormal brainstem auditory evoked potentials with normal inner ear function, may lead to improved detection and prevention of neurologic dysfunction and damage from bilirubin [22]. However, the exact mechanism for the described pathogenesis of bilirubin toxicity has never been clarified.

Here, the author tries to explain this finding based on the nanomaterial composition of blood brain barrier. First the author found out for the pore sizes of blood brain barrier in preterm and term neonate. According to the search, the pore sizes of blood brain barrier in preterm and term neonate are 1.2 nm and 0.8 nm [23–24], respectively. Then the author further reviewed for the sizes of conjugated and unconjugated bilirubin. According to the search, the sizes of conjugated and unconjugated bilirubin are 2.2 nm and 1 nm respectively [25].

Basically, passing thorough a pore, the molecule must have a smaller size than pore size of the membrane. Concerning the diffusion, at the controlled temperature and other environmental factors, conjugated bilirubin is unable to pass across blood brain barrier pore of neither preterm nor term neonate. While unconjugated bilirubin is able to pass across blood brain barrier of preterm but not term neonate. This can be a good explanation that the kernicterus is more common in preterm neonate and the cause is usually due to the unconjugated hyperbilirubinemia such as hemolysis.

JAUNDICE AND TOXICITY OF BILIRUBIN

Erythrocyte morphological changes have been seen with incubation of cells with different molar ratios of unconjugated bilirubin [26]. These changes occur as the bilirubin/human serum albumin molar ratio increases [26], This indicates that bilirubin can illicit toxicity in the erythrocyte membrane in a concentration and temperature-dependent manner [26]. Neonatal hyperbilirubinemia results from a predisposition to the production of unconjugated bilirubin in newborn infants and their limited ability to)conjugate it or(excrete it..Neonatal jaundice is a yellowing of the skin and eyeballs and may lead to deposition of bilirubin in brain cells [27]. Normally bilirubin is bound)conjugated(by a transport molecule and excreted [27]. However "unconjugated" bilirubin can induce a loss of neurons and atrophy of involved fiber systems, called kernicterus. Jaundice has become one of the most common problems in the neonatal period, which is not restricted to premature infants)< 37 weeks gestation([27].

Bilirubin can enter the brain if it is not bound to albumin or is unconjugated or if there has been damage to the blood brain barrier [28]. Once inside the brain, precipitation of bilirubin at low pH may have toxic effects [28]. Neurons undergoing differentiation are particularly susceptible to injury from bilirubin, suggesting that prematurity predisposes infants to bilirubin encaphalopathy [28]. It is necessary that the physiological and pathological jaundice should be differentiated. For normal or physiological jaundice [29], elevated unconjugated bilirubin can be observed. Total bilirubin generally peaks at 6-5 mg/dL on day 4-3 and then declines to adult levels by day 10. Asian infants usually peak at higher values 10) mg/dL(. For abnormal process, there are two groups: benign (breastmilk jaundice) and severe (pathological jaundice). For breast milk jaundice, elevated unconjugated bilirubin can be seen. Prolongation of physiologic jaundice is usually detected [30]. It is noted that 6%6 of breastfed babies jaundiced into 3rd week of life and may persist up to 3 months [30]. The pattern of neonatal jaundice is equivalent to starvation jaundice in adults. It should be noted that breastmilk jaundice can be divided into two types. The first type is early onset breastfeeding jaundice which may result from caloric deprivation and/or insufficient frequency of feeding [30]. This type of jaundice can be prevented or treated by encouraging mothers to nurse as frequently as possible, particularly if the bilirubin level is rising [30]. The second type is later onset, prolonged jaundice, known as the breast milk jaundice syndrome which is associated with one or more abnormalities in the maternal milk itself [30]. Concerning pathological jaundice, the jaundice is usually in 1st 24 hours and rapidly rising total bilirubin)> 5 mg/dL per day (can be seen and total bilirubin usually exceeds 17 mg/dL. The details of the common pathological steps for pathological jaundice can be seen in previous section.

Premature infants have higher rates of bilirubin production than do full term infants or adults because their red blood cells have a higher turnover rate and shorter life span [31]. Premature infants are also at increased risk of oxidative stress from hypoxia due to the immaturity of the lungs, followed by risk of hyperoxia once mechanical ventilation proceeds [31]. Infants are often exposed to oxygen concentrations as high as %95 [31]. For the premature infant, bilirubin has always been considered a toxin [32]. More recently bilirubin's antioxidant properties have been characterized [32]. It is possible therefore, that elevated bilirubin is an attempt by an immature fetus to cope with increased exposure to ROS [32]. Friel et al said that serum bilirubin in neonates correlated with total antioxidant activity [33].

For diagnosis of neonatal jaundice, the hyperbilirubinemia must be confirmed by the laboratory investigation. The basic clinical chemistry technique should be used. For alternative method, the physical examination can be used. If the bilirubin exceeds 5 mg/dL.

Caudal progression generally signifies higher total bilirubin levels. It should be noted that it should not rely on this system. Another new alternative is the used of transcutaneous analyzer. It is generally within 2 $\pm$ mg/dL of serum test and it is most useful if serum total bilirubin is less than 15 mg/dL [34]. The electronic device is proved to be useful when used as a screening method for identifying newborns who needed a serum bilirubin determination

[34]. Newer devices can be used not only as screening tools but also as reliable substitutes for serum bilirubin measurements [34].

For treatment of neonatal jaundice, 2004 AAP Guidelines should be followed [35]. Briefly, the early neonatal (before 72 hours) usually reflect severe pathology and required intensive care. For treatment, the phototherapy should be the first line choice. Special blue tube with light in blue-green spectrum is used. The lamp must be placed to infant and expose maximum surface area. If phototherapy is not successful, the exchange transfusion is recommended. Exchange transfusion removes bilirubin and antibodies from circulation. It is most beneficial to infants with hemolysis.

REFERENCES

[1] Tomaro ML, Batlle AM del C. Bilirubin: its role in cytoprotection against oxidative stress. *Int J Biol Cell Biol.* 2002; 34:216-220.

[2] Bizzarro MJ, Colson E, Ehrenkranz RA. Differential diagnosis and management of anemia in the newborn. *Pediatr Clin North Am.* 2004 Aug;51(4):1087-107, xi.

[3] Glader BE. Hemolytic anemia in children. *Clin Lab Med.* 1999 Mar;19(1):87-111, vi.

[4] Itoh S, Onishi S. Neonatal jaundice, hereditary hemolytic anemia. *Ryoikibetsu Shokogun Shirizu.* 1998; (19 Pt 2):251-8.

[5] Ahlfors CE, Wennberg RP. Bilirubin-albumin binding and neonatal jaundice. *Semin Perinatol.* 2004 Oct;28(5):334-9.

[6] Robertson A, Karp W, Brodersen R. Bilirubin displacing effect of drugs used in neonatology. *Acta Paediatr Scand.* 1991 Dec;80(12):1119-27.

[7] Brodersen R, Friis-Hansen B, Stern L.Drug-induced displacement of bilirubin from albumin in the newborn. *Dev Pharmacol Ther.* 1983; 6(4):217-29.

[8] Shevell MI, Majnemer A, Schiff D. Neurologic perspectives of Crigler-Najjar syndrome type I. *J Child Neurol.* 1998 Jun;13(6):265-9.

[9] Wiwanitkit V. Gilbert's syndrome: a case report. *Med J Ubon Hosp* 2000; 21: 209-211.

[10] Mammaev SN. Molecular diagnosis of heritable unconjugated hyperbilirubinemias. *Klin Lab Diagn.* 2005 Dec;(12):8-13.

[11] Wiwanitkit V. Laboratory investigation in neonatal jaundice. *Med J Ubon Hosp* 2001; 22: 231 – 9.

[12] Wiwanitkit V. High serum alkaline phosphatase levels, a study in 181 Thai adult hospitalized patients. *BMC Fam Pract.* 2001; 2:2.

[13] Gupta R, Nagdeve NG, Sarin YK. Neonatal surgical jaundice revisited. *Indian J Pediatr.* 2005 May;72(5):415-23.

[14] Wiwanitkit V. Energy change in the formation of conjugated bilirubin: A possible responsive mechanism for liver cell pathology. *Rev Esp Enferm Dig.* 2007 Feb;99(2):94-95.

[15] Seyfried H, Klicpera M, Leithner C, Penner E. Bilirubin metabolism (author's transl). *Wien Klin Wochenschr.* 1976; 88:477-82.

[16] Adachi Y, Kobayashi H, Shouji M, Kitano M, Okuyama Y, Yamamoto T. Functional integrity of hepatocyte canalicular membrane transport of taurocholate and bilirubin diglucuronide in Eisai hyperbilirubinuria rats. *Life Sci.* 1993; 52:777-84.
[17] Granato A, Gores G, Vilei MT, Tolando R, Ferraresso C, Muraca M. Bilirubin inhibits bile acid induced apoptosis in rat hepatocytes. *Gut.* 2003; 52:1774-8.
[18] Shapiro SM. 2003. Bilirubin toxicity in the developing nervous system. *Pediatr Neurol, 29*:410-21.
[19] Wiwanitkit V. 2006. Neonatal Jaundice. 46th Annual conference of the Indian Society of Haematology and Transfusion medicine. Imphal, Manipur on 14th to 16th January 2006
[20] Truman P. 2006. Jaundice in the preterm infant. *Paediatr Nurs, 18*:20-2.
[21] Juretschke LJ. 2005. Kernicterus: still a concern. *Neonatal Netw, 24*:7-19.
[22] Shapiro SM, Bhutani VK, Johnson L. 2006. Hyperbilirubinemia and kernicterus. *Clin Perinatol, 33*:387-410.
[23] Calhoun DA, Murthy SN, Bryant BG, Luedtke SA, Bhatt-Mehta V. 2006. Recent advances in neonatal pharmacotherapy. *Ann Pharmacother, 40*:710-9.
[24] van Bree JB, de Boer AG, Danhof M, Ginsel LA, Breimer DD. 1988. Characterization of an "in vitro" blood-brain barrier: effects of molecular size and lipophilicity on cerebrovascular endothelial transport rates of drugs. *J Pharmacol Exp Ther, 247*:1233-9.
[25] Seyfried H, Klicpera M, Leithner C, Penner E. Bilirubin metabolism. *Wien Klin Wochenschr.* 1976; 88:477-82.
[26] Brito MA, Silva R, Tiribelli C, Brites D. Assessment of bilirubin toxicity to erythrocytes. Implication in neonatal jaundice management. *European J Clinical Invest.* 2000; 30: 239-247.
[27] Gurses D, Kilic I, Sahiner T. Effects of hyperbilirubinemia on cerebrocortical electrical activity in newborns. *Pediatr Res.* 2002; 52:125-130.
[28] Dennery PA, Seidman DS, Stevenson DK. Neonatal Hyperbilirubinemi. *New Engl J Med* 2001; 344: 581-590.
[29] Blackburn S. Hyperbilirubinemia and neonatal jaundice. *Neonatal Netw.* 1995 Oct;14(7):15-25.
[30] Leung AK, Sauve RS. Breastfeeding and breast milk jaundice. *J R Soc Health.* 1989 Dec;109(6):213-7.
[31] Friel JK, Martin SM, Langdon M, Herzberg G, Buettner GR. Human milk provides better antioxidant protection than does infant formula. *Pediatr Res.* 2002; 51;612-618.
[32] Hansen TWR. Bilirubin production, breast-feeding and neonatal jaundice. *Acta Paediatrica.* 2001; 90:716-723.
[33] Friel J,Widness J, Jiang T, Belkhode SL, Rebouche CJ, Ziegler EE. Antioxidant status and oxidant stress are associated with vitamin E intakes in VLBW infants in early life. *Nutr Res* 2002; 22:55-64.
[34] Bertini G, Rubaltelli FF. Non-invasive bilirubinometry in neonatal jaundice. *Semin Neonatol.* 2002 Apr;7(2):129-33.
[35] Subcommittee on Hyperbilirubinemia. Management of hyperbilirubinemia in the newborn infant. *Pediatrics* 2004; 114;297-316.

Chapter 3

CORD BLOOD BANKING AND CELL THERAPY

INTRODUCTION TO UMBILICAL CORD

Umbilical cord is the organ that connects to the placenta and fetus's body. It is the way that blood from mother passes to the fetus. Cord blood is the blood remaining in the umbilical cord of a baby after the baby's birth [1]. This blood has been found to have some special characteristics and is found to be a rich source of stem cells, which generate the blood cells in our body [1]. Basically, fetal cardiac output is high, and the heart has not been shown to have the sustained reserves demonstrated in the adult heart. About 40% (of the combined output of both ventricles (CVO) is directed to the umbilical circulation [2]. Hypoxaemia, acidaemia and various vasomotor agents influence the partition of cardiac output between systemic and umbilical circulations, with or without relatively small changes of blood pressure, which is low by adult standards [2]. In general, the conductance of systemic circuits is more susceptible to change than that of the umbilical [2]. The ductus venosus, which is situated within the liver parenchyma, is a vascular shunt unique to the fetal and neonatal circulations [3]. In fetal life, the ductus venosus allows variable portions of the umbilical and portal venous blood flows to bypass the liver microcirculation [3]. After birth, when the umbilical circulation ceases, blood flow through the ductus venosus decreases substantially [3]. Generally, the umbilical circulation under physiological conditions is protected by the amniotic fluid [4]. This protective mechanism of the amniotic fluid may be disturbed artificially or spontaneously by the rupture of the membranes [4]. Circulating hematopoietic stem and progenitor cells play important roles in the physiology and homeostasis of the hematopoietic system [5]. The frequency of these cells varies throughout development, being more abundant during gestation [5]. During the last two decades, circulating cells of newborns presenting in umbilical cord blood has gained relevance not only because of their biology, but also because of their clinical application [5].

The umbilical cord is the lifeline of the fetus and of the neonate in the first few minutes after birth [6]. Care of the cord and stump in the immediate neonatal period varies according to social, cultural, economic, and geographic factors [6]. Measures taken to insure sterility in cutting, tying, and painting the umbilical cord may prevent serious diseases such as tetanus neonatorum [6]. In addition to the general umbilical care, now the procedure on cord blood sampling is the new emerging useful technique for novel stem cell therapy. In this chapter, the details on cord blood banking and cell therapy will be focused.

Cord Blood Collection

A. General Introduction

After a baby's birth, once the umbilical cord is clamped, a small amount of residual blood remains in the umbilical cord [1]. This is collected into a special blood bag and then taken for storing and processing [1]. As the collection of the umbilical cord blood happens after the baby's birth, it does not affect the baby's birth and also no harm is caused to the baby or the mother [1,7]. A well-accepted use of cord blood is as an alternative to bone marrow as a source of hematopoietic stem cells for allogeneic transplantation to siblings or to unrelated recipients; women can donate cord blood for unrelated recipients to public banks [8-9]. However, the emerging medical ethics problem in cord blood collection is the commercial cord blood banking [10-11]. According to the Working Group on Ethical Issues in Umbilical Cord Blood Banking, umbilical cord blood banking for autologous use is associated with even greater uncertainty than banking for allogeneic use, marketing practices for umbilical cord blood banking in the private sector need close attention and the process of obtaining informed consent for collection of umbilical cord blood should begin before labor and delivery [11].

Since 1988, allogeneic cord blood transplantations have been used in the hematology and oncology area [12]. Cord blood banks, either public or from non-profit corporations, opened in several countries Umbilical cord blood can be collected and stored frozen for years [8].

B. Cord Blood Collection Procedure

Cord blood collection should be undertaken within a total quality system and good manufacturing practice facilities. Protocols should be developed based upon risk assessment and cost efficiency [13]. It is recommended that cord blood collection should be after the permission for cord blood donation [14]. Surbek et al reported a high acceptance of umbilical cord blood donation for banking and stem cell transplantation purposes in pregnant women, irrespective of previous knowledge [15]. As there are no major differences between women of different ethnic background, a high degree of diversity of HLA-types of donated cord blood samples can be expected and may offset the underrepresentation of ethnic minorities in bone marrow donor registries [15]. Danzer et al reported a high degree of satisfaction of unrelated umbilical cord blood donation for banking in women 6 months after delivery [16]. Despite a well-performed and detailed informed consent procedure, one of the ongoing issues for the donators in cord blood banking involves the concern regarding of improper use of the cells, such as genetic testing or experimentation [16]. Accurate and detailed counseling of pregnant women and their partners therefore maximizes the likelihood that they will donate cord blood for unrelated banking.

For cord blood collection, there are 3 common: Method 1 = Hanging method after delivering the placenta, Method 2 = Aspiration from in utero placenta, Method 3 = Aspiration from in utero placenta and Syringe-assisted aspiration. Wacharaprechanont et al recently performed a comparative study on the 3 methods using the closed system and showed that method 3 was the best method but it required more trained personnel and involved a complicated procedure [17]. After collection, the quality of the cord blood (volume, total white blood cells (WBC) count, CD34+ and sterility control) must be checked. According to a recent study from Thailand, the quality of the cord blood collected by any methods was satisfactory and discard rate of collecting units were comparable with data reported from other cord blood banks [17]. However, Wong et al found that the reduction of stem and progenitor cells correlated significantly with that of major cell populations, indicating a general cell loss, possibly due to clotting activities developed with time [18]. They documented strong evidence for recommending the collection of cord blood before the delivery of the placenta [19]. At present, the ex utero collection is more widely used. Basically, the umbilical vein is punctured or catheterized, and then placental/cord blood is aspirated with syringes contained anticoagulants [20]. Another method is to drain blood into a collection-bag by gravity [20]. The collection bags with anticoagulants are manufactured by TERUMO and BAXTER HEALTHCARE CO [20]. Askari et al said that donor selection and collection technique modifications might improve product quality [21]. They noted that total nucleated cell count appeared to be more affected by different variables than CD34+ count [21].

Table 1. Methods for cord blood collection

Methods	Details
1. Hanging method after delivering the placenta	The umbilical cord blood is collected after the placenta is delivered [18]. The entire collection process takes places after the umbilical cord is clamped off from the newborn [18]. The placenta is then placed into a sterile device with the umbilical cord hanging through [18]. The cord blood is collected by draining the cord blood with the help of gravity [18]. In this case, they can usually collect between 40 and 150 milliliters of blood [18].
2. Aspiration from in utero placenta	The cord blood is collected from the umbilical vein with 20-mL syringes while the placenta was in utero.
3. Aspiration from in utero placenta and Syringe-assisted aspiration	The collection of cord blood involved direct aspiration via puncture of the ethanol-sterilized umbilical vein at a site distal to the placenta, to reduce to a minimum the possibility of cross-contamination by maternal lymphocyte.

Blood Banking for Cord Blood

To establish a cord blood bank large panels of frozen, HLA-typed cord blood units need to be stored. Cryopreserved, unprocessed cord blood units require vast storage space. Various procedures can be used to isolate stem and progenitor cells from cord blood to reduce the volume of blood. The described methods include hydroxyethyl starch sedimentation (HES) with two centrifugation steps, and the top and bottom (T&B) isolation of buffy coat following a single centrifugation, and filter systems for processing cord blood (such as those developed by Asahi Kasei Medical and Terumo: Procord). The hydroxyethyl starch method and the T & B method have been used worldwide for the volume reduction of human placental/umbilical cord blood units [22]. The new filter system was shown to be efficient for placenta cord blood processing, encompassing a very simple handling procedure with a good recovery of haematopoietic progenitor cells [22]. Takahashi et al indicated that filters that capture stem and progenitor cells might be an appropriate methodology for processing cord blood collected for banking [23]. Dal Cortivo et al proposed that Procord was an efficient method for erythrocyte depletion of cord blood, and recoveries of nucleated cells and progenitor cells are comparable to those obtained with similar processing [23]. Nevertheless, as all existing methods, it is associated with cell and progenitor cell loss [24]. At present, automated system for reduction of blood volume is also applied. Armitage et al studied using the Optipress II Automated Blood Component Extractor (Opti II) from Baxter Healthcare Corporation, to reduce the volume of the cord blood collection, preserving the quantity and quality of the progenitor cells, in a closed system [25]. They reported that using this method for processing cord blood units reduced storage requirement by two-thirds but preserves the quantity and quality of the progenitor cells [25]. Solves et al recently compared two different methods for CB volume reduction in both development and routine phases: HES sedimentation and T & B fractionation with the Optipress II [26]. According to this work, the volume reduction method with the Optipress II was a time-saving system that allows good cell recoveries [26]. In contrast, the main advantage of the HES method is the higher RBC depletion that influences CFU content. Reducing RBC content must be the object of further improvements for volume reduction using the Optipress II method [26].

Although placental blood has recently become a new source of hematopoietic progenitors for marrow replacement, limited attention has been given to systems suitable to ensure the short-term and long-term quality of placental blood units used for transplantation [27]. For cord blood banking, quality system is needed [27 - 28]. It includes the organizational structure, procedures, processes and resources needed to implement quality management [27-28]. The number of cord blood banks throughout the world is increasing rapidly [29]. In the USA and Europe, more than ten thousans placental cord blood units are stored and available for transplantation [29]. The practices of umbilical cord blood collection, mother selection, infectious disease screening, cell manipulation and storage must be standardized [29]. Some accreditation process should be mandatory for assessing operating procedures and the quality assurance programs of the banks, and for allowing the international exchange of placental blood between transplant centers. Medical ISOs can be applied [27-28]. The Quality System must be maintained and subjected to external audit at regular intervals so that certification is confirmed [27-28].

CORD BLOOD THERAPY

A. Cord Blood Transfusion

Autologous cord blood transfusion can be seen in medical practice [30]. Ballin et al said that blood collected from the umbilical cord was a safe source for autotransfusion, provided that bacteriological testing has been carried out [31]. Imura et al proposed that autologous cord-blood transfusion had the potential to be a useful alternative to homologous transfusion in newborns requiring surgery [32]. Adequate collection and storage techniques for cord-blood must be developed [32]. For the procedure, the umbilical vein is pierced with an 18-gauge needle, and placental blood is withdrawn into two 50-ml syringes filled with 4 ml of citrate-phosphate-dextrose solution. Autologous transfusion with packed red cells obtained from autologous cord blood can be used for surgery [32-33]. Tagushi et al concluded that autologous cord blodo transfusion was considered beneficial because it enabled neonatal surgical patients to avoid allotransfusions, therefore, autologous cord-blood storage should be considered in the patients antenatally diagnosed to have surgical malformations [34]. However, the storage volume varies for each case, therefore, improved techniques to obtain an adequate amount of blood also should be developed [34]. Conclusively, autologous cord blood transfusion is the new advancement in transfusion medicine for neonate.

B. Cord Blood Transplantation

Cord blood transplantation is widely used as an alternative to bone marrow transplantation at present. Over the last decade, umbilical cord blood has become a viable option for hematopoietic stem cell transplants. The literature shows that after umbilical cord blood transplantation the relapse rate, disease-free survival and overall survival of patients with myeloid malignancies is similar to other hematopoietic stem cells sources [35]. Disease status at the time of transplantation is found in several studies to be a very important determinant of long-term outcome [35]. Brunstein et al said that umbilical cord blood was a valuable alternative source of hematopoietic stem cells for transplantation of patients with myeloid malignancies who required an allogeneic transplant, but lack a suitable sibling donor [35]. The number of umbilical cord blood transplants is increasing worldwide. Gluckman reported that engraftment with cord blood was delayed resulting in an increased incidence of early transplant complications [36]. Gluckman also reported that the incidence of acute and chronic graft-vs-host disease was reduced with cord blood grafts even in HLA-mismatched transplants and in adults [36]. The option of performing cord blood transplants should be based on urgency of the transplant, cord blood cell dose and number of HLA disparities [37].

Cord blood transplants have a favorably low risk of graft-versus-host disease even in mismatched transplants [38]. Stem cell dose is an independent factor in transplants from any source, determining engraftment, transplant-related mortality and risk of leukemic relapse [38]. Indeed, graft cell dose is an important determinant of hematopoietic recovery and overall outcome following umbilical cord blood transplantation, and the limited cell dose of single umbilical cord blood units has been a major barrier to its more widespread use [39]. A limiting factor has been the 10-fold lower cell dose in a cord blood unit compared with harvested bone marrow or peripheral blood stem cells [40]. The low cell dose leads to delayed engraftment and an increase in graft failure [40]. The use of umbilical cord blood in older children and adult patients has been limited by the fixed, low cell dose available in a umbilical cord blood unit, relative to recipient weight. This can be overcome by strategies such as using two or more umbilical cord blood units [41]. Transplantation with two unrelated umbilical cord blood units is feasible, safe and effective and can overcome the limitation of cell dose of single umbilical cord blood units [39-41].

Stem Cell Therapy

With the isolation of human embryonic stem cells (hESCs) in 1998 came the realization of a long-sought aspiration for an unlimited source of human tissue. hESCs theoretically represent an unlimited supply of normal differentiated cells to engineer diseased tissues to regain normal function [42]. However, before hESCs can be useful as human therapeutics, technologies must be developed to provide them with the specific signals required to differentiate in a controlled fashion, to regulate and/or shut down the growth of hESCs and their progeny once they have been transferred to the recipient, and to circumvent the recognition of non-autologous hESC-derived cells as foreign [42]. The methods for deriving hESCs are well established and repeatable and are relatively successful with a ratio of 1:10 to 1:2 new hESC lines produced from 4- to 8-d-old morula and blastocysts and from isolated inner cell mass cell clusters of human blastocysts [43]. The hESCs can be formed and maintained on human somatic cells in humanized serum-free culture conditions and for several passages in cell-free culture systems. The hESCs can be transfected with DNA constructs [43]. hESCs spontaneously differentiate in the absence of the appropriate cell feeder layer, when overgrown in culture and when isolated from the ESC colony [43]. All three major embryonic lineages are produced in differentiating flat attachment cultures and unattached embryoid bodies [43]. Cell progenitors of interest can be identified by markers, expression of reporter genes, and characteristic morphology, and the cells thereafter enriched for progenitor types and further culture to more mature cell types [43]. hESC represent a theoretically inexhaustible source of precursor cells that could be differentiated into any cell type to treat degenerative, malignant, or genetic diseases, or injury due to inflammation, infection, and trauma [44]. This pluripotent, endlessly dividing cell has been hailed as a possible means for treating diabetes, Parkinson's disease, Alzheimer's, spinal cord injury, heart failure, and bone marrow failure [44]. The difficulty of differentiating ESCs to pure, clinically exploitable cell populations to treat genetic and degenerative diseases is being solved in part with the help of genetically modified cell lines [45]. With progress in genome editing and somatic cell nuclear transfer, it is theoretically possible to obtain genetically repaired isogenic cells [45]. Moreover, the prospect of being able to select, isolate and expand a single cell to a vast population of cells could achieve a unique level of quality control, until now unattainable in the field of gene therapy [45]. Stem cell technology plus gene therapy is the new hope for treatment of present untreatable diseases.

REFERENCES

[1] What is Cord Blood? Available online at www.cordbloodbankingguide.com

[2] Mott JC. Control of the foetal circulation. *J Exp Biol.* 1982 Oct;100:129-46.

[3] Edelstone DI. Regulation of blood flow through the ductus venosus. *J Dev Physiol.* 1980 Aug;2(4):219-38.

[4] Kunzel W. Umbilical circulation--physiology and pathology. *J Perinat Med.* 1981;9 Suppl 1:68-71.

[5] Mayani H, Alvarado-Moreno JA, Flores-Guzman P. Biology of human hematopoietic stem and progenitor cells present in circulation. *Arch Med Res.* 2003 Nov-Dec;34(6):476-88.

[6] Elhassani SB. The umbilical cord: care, anomalies, and diseases. *South Med J.* 1984 Jun;77(6):730-6.

[7] Fyle J. Routine commercial umbilical cord blood collection. *RCM Midwives.* 2006 Jul;9(7):261.

[8] Fisk NM, Roberts IA, Markwald R, Mironov V. Can routine commercial cord blood banking be scientifically and ethically justified? *PLoS Med.* 2005 Feb;2(2):e44.

[9] Drew D. Umbilical cord blood banking. *Adv Nurse Pract.* 2005 Apr;13(4):Suppl 2-6

[10] Kusminsky G. Umbilical cord blood criopreservation for autologous use. An ethical problem. *Medicina (B Aires).* 2006;66(4):367-71.

[11] Sugarman J, Kaalund V, Kodish E, Marshall MF, Reisner EG, Wilfond BS, Wolpe PR. Ethical issues in umbilical cord blood banking. Working Group on Ethical Issues in Umbilical Cord Blood Banking. *JAMA.* 1997 Sep 17;278(11):938-43.

[12] Dalle JH. Cord blood banking: public versus private banks--facts to ponder and consider. *Arch Pediatr.* 2005 Mar;12(3):298-304.

[13] Warwick RM, Barbara JA. Safety aspects of cord blood banking. *Bone Marrow Transplant.* 1998 Jun;21 Suppl 3:S40-2.

[14] Kommission Qualitatssicherung der Schweizerischen Gesellschaft fur Gynakologie und Geburtshilfe. Umbilical cord blood donation: unrelated donation, familial (directed) donation and autologous donation (private banking) *Gynakol Geburtshilfliche Rundsch.* 2003 Apr;43(2):118-21.

[15] Surbek DV, Islebe A, Schonfeld B, Tichelli A, Gratwohl A, Holzgreve W. Umbilical cord blood transplantation: acceptance of umbilical cord blood donation by pregnant patients. *Schweiz Med Wochenschr.* 1998 May 2;128(18):689-95

[16] Danzer E, Holzgreve W, Troeger C, Kostka U, Steimann S, Bitzer J, Gratwohl A, Tichelli A, Seelmann K, Surbek DV. Attitudes of Swiss mothers toward unrelated umbilical cord blood banking 6 months after donation. *Transfusion.* 2003 May;43(5):604-8.

[17] Wacharaprechanont T, O-Charoen R, Vanichsetakul P, Sudjai D, Kupatawintu P, Seksarn P, Samritpradit P, Charoenvidhya D. Cord blood collection for the National Cord Blood Bank in Thailand. *J Med Assoc Thai.* 2003 Jun;86 Suppl 2:S409-16.

[18] Cord blood collection. Available online at http://www.cordplan.com/en/cord-blood-collection.html

[19] Wong A, Yuen PM, Li K, Yu AL, Tsoi WC. Cord blood collection before and after placental delivery: levels of nucleated cells, haematopoietic progenitor cells, leukocyte subpopulations and macroscopic clots. *Bone Marrow Transplant.* 2001 Jan;27(2):133-8.

[20] Ohnuma K, Nishihira H. Harvest techniques for cord blood after delivery of placenta. *Rinsho Byori.* 1999 May;Suppl 110:21-7.

[21] Askari S, Miller J, Chrysler G, McCullough J. Impact of donor- and collection-related variables on product quality in ex utero cord blood banking. *Transfusion.* 2005 Feb;45(2):189-94.

[22] Yasutake M, Sumita M, Terashima S, Tokushima Y, Nitadori Y, Takahashi TA. Stem cell collection filter system for human placental/umbilical cord blood processing. *Vox Sang.* 2001 Feb;80(2):101

[23] Takahashi TA, Rebulla P, Armitage S, van Beckhoven J, Eichler H, Kekomaki R, Letowska M, Wahab F, Moroff G. Multi-laboratory evaluation of procedures for reducing the volume of cord blood: influence on cell recoveries. *Cytotherapy.* 2006;8(3):254-64.

[24] Dal Cortivo L, Robert I, Mangin C, Sameshima T, Kora S, Gluckman E, Benbunan M, Marolleau JP. Cord blood banking: volume reduction using "Procord" Terumo filter. *J Hematother Stem Cell Res.* 2000 Dec;9(6):885-90.

[25] Armitage S, Fehily D, Dickinson A, Chapman C, Navarrete C, Contreras M. Cord blood banking: volume reduction of cord blood units using a semi-automated closed system. *Bone Marrow Transplant.* 1999 Mar;23(5):505-9.

[26] Solves P, Mirabet V, Planelles D, Blasco I, Perales A, Carbonell-Uberos F, Soler MA, Roig R. Red blood cell depletion with a semiautomated system or hydroxyethyl starch sedimentation for routine cord blood banking: a comparative study. Transfusion. 2005 Jun;45(6):867-73.

[27] Sirchia G, Rebulla P, Lecchi L, Mozzi F, Crepaldi R, Parravicini A. Implementation of a quality system (ISO 9000 series) for placental blood banking. *J Hematother.* 1998 Feb;7(1):19-35.

[28] Sirchia G, Rebulla P, Mozzi F, Lecchi L, Lazzari L, Ratti I. A quality system for placental blood banking. *Bone Marrow Transplant.* 1998 Jun;21 Suppl 3:S43-7.

[29] Traineau R, Dal Cortivo L. Cord blood banks--unrelated transplants. *Transfus Clin Biol.* 1998 Feb;5(1):56-63.

[30] Balin A, Kenet G. Autologous cord blood transfusion. *Harefua*h. 1993 May 2;124(9):554-6.

[31] Ballin A, Arbel E, Kenet G, Berar M, Kohelet D, Tanay A, Zakut H, Meytes D. Autologous umbilical cord blood transfusion. *Arch Dis Child Fetal Neonatal* Ed. 1995 Nov;73(3):F181-3.

[32] Imura K, Kawahara H, Kitayama Y, Yoneda A, Yagi M, Suehara N. Usefulness of cord-blood harvesting for autologous transfusion in surgical newborns with antenatal diagnosis of congenital anomalies. *J Pediatr Surg.* 2001 Jun;36(6):851-4.

[33] Hosono S, Mugishima H, Nakano Y, Murabayashi M, Shimada M, Minato M, Takahashi S, Harada K, Ikeda T, Fukuzawa M. Autologous cord blood transfusion in an infant with a huge sacrococcygeal teratoma. *J Perinat Med.* 2004;32(2):187-9.

[34] Taguchi T, Suita S, Nakamura M, Yamanouchi T, Ogita K, Taguchi S, Uesugi T, Nakano H, Inaba S. The efficacy of autologous cord-blood transfusions in neonatal surgical patients. *J Pediatr Surg.* 2003 Apr;38(4):604-7.

[35] Brunstein CG, Baker KS, Wagner JE. Umbilical cord blood transplantation for myeloid malignancies. *Curr Opin Hematol.* 2007 Mar;14(2):162-9.

[36] Gluckman E. Current status of umbilical cord blood hematopoietic stem cell transplantation. *Exp Hematol.* 2000 Nov;28(11):1197-205.

[37] Gluckman E, Rocha V. Cord blood transplant: strategy of alternative donor search. *Springer Semin Immunopathol.* 2004 Nov;26(1-2):143-54.

[38] Schmitz N, Barrett J. Optimizing engraftment--source and dose of stem cells. *Semin Hematol.* 2002 Jan;39(1):3-14.

[39] Majhail NS, Brunstein CG, Wagner JE. Double umbilical cord blood transplantation. *Curr Opin Immunol.* 2006 Oct;18(5):571-5.

[40] Haspel RL, Ballen KK. Double cord blood transplants: filling a niche? *Stem Cell Rev.* 2006;2(2):81-6.

[41] O'Brien TA, Tiedemann K, Vowels MR. No longer a biological waste product: umbilical cord blood. *Med J Aust.* 2006 Apr 17;184(8):407-10.

[42] Strulovici Y, Leopold PL, O'connor TP, Pergolizzi RG, Crystal RG. Human Embryonic Stem Cells and Gene Therapy. *Mol Ther.* 2007 Mar 13;

[43] Trounson A. The production and directed differentiation of human embryonic stem cells. *Endocr Rev.* 2006 Apr;27(2):208-19.

[44] Lerou PH, Daley GQ. Therapeutic potential of embryonic stem cells. *Blood Rev.* 2005 Nov;19(6):321-31.

[45] Yates F, Daley GQ. Progress and prospects: gene transfer into embryonic stem cells. *Gene Ther.* 2006 Oct;13(20):1431-9.

Chapter 4

NEONATAL HEMATO-ONCOLOGY

INTRODUCTION

Malignant disorder is an important group of diseases with high mortality. Basically, malignancy is an uncontrolled growth of cell. This is common for geriatric population. Both genetic and environmental factors are quoted for their roles in carcinogeneis. However, malignancy can occur in all age group including to the neonate. Recent advances in genetic testing and studies of cohorts of cancer patients have demonstrated the likelihood of identifying a cancer susceptibility mutation for numerous childhood cancers [1]. Inherited predisposition to cancer is frequently the result of dominant constitutional mutations in tumor suppressor genes, which can be inherited from an affected parent or occur de novo during gametogenesis [1]. The well-known hematological cancer in the neonate is congenital leukemia. There are also other important cancer in the neonate, especially for "-blastoma" type malignancies. In this chapter, the details on the congenital leukemia and other important "-blastoma" type malignancies will be summarized and presented.

CONGENITAL LEUKEMIA

A. Introduction

Congenital leukemia is an important malignancy in the neonate. It is the malignancy of the white blood cells. Congenital leukemia is a defined as the leukemia diagnosed from birth to 6 weeks of age [2-3]. It is a very rare disease and its actual etiology is still unknown [2-3]. The association of some specific congenital syndromes with leukemia provides an opportunity to study the process of leukemogenesis on the background of known genetic alterations [3]. The role of the intracellular DNA damage response system in suppressing leukemia is demonstrated by the congenital disorders of genomic instability [3]. Congenital leukemia is mentioned for the association with Trisomy 7, Turner's syndrome and Mosaic trisomy 9 [2-3]. Slayton and Schibler noted that congenital bone marrow failure syndromes were associated with a number of congenital abnormalities affecting a wide range of organ systems and these syndromes predisposed patients to leukemia [4]. Further studies for the actual pathogenesis of congenital anemia are still needed.

Concerning the prevalence of congenital leukemia, it is sporadically reported in many countries. Less than 300 cases are documented in the literatures. Congenital leukemia is an important congenital malignancy. This disease was first described by Smith in 1921 and has been continuously reported [5]. Generally, Acute leukemias in infants, including the congenital and neonatal leukemia, present a number of unfavourable features [6]. Cvetkovic and Cvetkovic noted that age of the infant, hyperleukocytosis, outstanding organomegaly, early onset of the CNS leukemia were some of the factors causing this group of acute leukemias of childhood to be those with highest risk [6].

Concerning the clinical features of congenital anemia, the main clinical presentations include nodular skin infiltrates (leukemia cutis), hepatosplenomegaly, pallor, purpura or petechiae and respiratory distress. For diagnosis, multiparameter flow cytometry with optimally selected antibody combinations has expanded the use of this technique beyond traditional applications in hematopathology [7]. By analyzing qualitative patterns of antigen expression on discrete populations or "clusters," one can detect immunophenotypic aberrancy in specific cell populations relative to normal and reactive populations [7]. Evaluation of patterns of antigen expression can also be used to supplement conventional methodologies in the diagnosis and subclassification of certain types of hematologic neoplasia [7].

Of interest, there are evidences on the co-expression between some congenital syndromes and leukemia. The association of specific congenital syndromes with leukemia provides an opportunity to study the process of leukemogenesis on the background of known genetic alterations [8]. The role of the intracellular DNA damage response system in suppressing leukemia is demonstrated by the congenital disorders of genomic instability [8]. Specific collaborations between survival and differentiation pathways characterize the leukemias observed in Down, Noonan and neurofibromatosis syndromes [8].

B. Experience on Congenital Leukemia from Thailand

For Thailand, a Southeast Asian country, this leukemia is rare. In Thailand, the first report of congenital leukemia was reported by Ketusingh *et al* in 1962 [9]. The patient is a female preterm newborn with leukemia cutis [9]. Since the first case report, there have been seldom reports of congenital leukemia in Thailand. Here, the author retrospectively studied on the reports of congenital leukemia in Thailand in order to study the clinical summary of congenital leukemia among Thai patients. This study was designed as a descriptive retrospective study. A literature review of the papers concerning congenital leukemia in Thailand was performed, using the database of published works cited in the Index Medicus and Science Citation Index. The author also reviewed the published works in all 256 local Thai journals, which are not included in the international citation index, in the database "Thai Index Medicus" (161.200.96.233/thaiim.html). The literature review focused on the years 1962 - 2004. According to the literature review, reports were recruited for further study. The details of clinical presentations of the patients in all included papers were studied.

According to this study, there have been reports of at least 3 cases of congenital leukemia [9-11] (Table 1). Two of the three patients were detected in the day 1 after birth (range, 1 day – 23 days) with a male: female ratio of 2: 1. All cases were preterm newborns and had no other associated congenital disorder. Concerning the maternal history at pregnancy, only 1 case [5] had the risk history as gestational influenza. Concerning the clinical presentation, nodular skin infiltrates (leukemia cutis), hepatosplenomegaly and petchiae can be seen in 2 cases [9,11], 2 cases [9,11] and 1 case [10], respectively. Some unusual presentations as testicular swelling and abdominal distention can be seen in 1 case [10]. Concerning the laboratory investigation, the average for white blood count is 155,533.33 ± 127,684.04 cells/mm [4]. The type of leukemia are myeloid leukemia in 2 cases [9,11] and lymphoid leukemia in 1 case [10]. Concerning the treatment, no case got the specific chemotherapy. Of interest, 1 of 3 cases survived and diagnosed as remission. However, this case lost following up. Concerning the pathology from autopsies of the two lethal cases, the infiltration of leukemia cells in brains, lungs and hearts can be seen in both cases.

Table 1. Cases of congenital leukemia in the Thai literatures [9-11]

sex	Age at diagnosis	Clinical presentation	Laboratory investigations		Definitive diagnosis	treatment	outcome
			White blood count (cell/mm^3)	Immature cell (%)			
Female	1 day	Purplish skin nodules overall the body, hepatosplenomegaly.	57,800	promonocyte predominately (72 %)	Bone marrow study	No	Cure (within 2 months)
Female	1 day	Purplish skin nodules overall the body, hepatosplenomegaly.	300,000	lymphoblast prominately (20 %)	Autopsy	Blood transfusion, steroid, antibiotic	died (at the age of 40 days)
Male	23 days	Petichiae, abdominal distention, testicular swelling	108,800	myeloblast prominately (53 %)	Autopsy	no	died (at the age of 2 days)

In this study, the leukemia cutis and hepatosplenomegaly are the two most common presentations (66.67 %). Resnik and Brod noted that leukemia cutis was rarely reported in the dermatology literature despite various authors citing 50% of infants with congenital leukemia had skin involvement [12]. They found that specific cutaneous leukemic infiltrates occurred in 25% to 30% of infants with congenital leukemia and usually appear as firm blue, red, or purple nodules in a generalized distribution [12]. They also notified that although the high incidence of gingival and oral infiltrates was reported in adult monocytic leukemia, only 1% of congenital leukemia patients had oral involvement [12]. According to this study, the skin lesion appeared all over the patients' bodies as well. Similar to the finding of Resnik and Brod [12], leukemia cutis does not alter the clinical course of congenital leukemia. OF interest, some uncommon presentations of congenital leukemia as abdominal distention and testicular swelling can be seen in this series.

Concerning the maternal risk history, no predominant risk can be identified. In addition, no associated congenital disorder can be seen in any case. However, all cases in this study has been documented for a long time and the cytogenetic study was not available at that time. Recently, Bresters *et al* performed the cytogenetic study for the congenital leukemia and noted that cytogenetic abnormalities were found in the majority of the patients tested (72%); 11q23 abnormalities were found in less than half of them (42%) [13]. All cases in this study present severe leukocytosis. Considering the type of leukemia in this study, myeloid is more frequent than lymphoid. This finding is similar to that of Bresters *et al* [10].

Concerning treatment, no case got proper chemotherapy. This is according to the fact that these cases were managed in the period that no effective chemotherapy was available. However, a remission can be seen in 1 case [9]. This case had got no treatment because the parents refused. In this case, the patient was still alive without any abnormality at 2 months. Unluckily, no more data on the following can be derived. Bresters *et al* said that in the patients at risk, the probability of event-free survival (EFS) and disease-free survival (DFS) were significantly higher in myeloid than in lymphoid leukemia and 8 % of the patients with congenital myeloid leukemia could had spontaneous remissions [13].

Conclusively, the author found that the congenital leukemia is very rare in Thailand. The pattern of clinical presentation and clinical course of disease are similar to other reports. However, some interesting presentations can be seen. Due to the fact that all cases were diagnosed in the period that the effective chemotherapy is available, no proper treatment was prescribed. Of interest, the spontaneous remission can be seen in this study. An interesting question due to this retrospective study is the null incidence of leukemia in the recent two decades despite the more advanced diagnostic technology in Thailand. This finding might reflex to the better antenatal care, better perinatal screening and better self care of the pregnant to lower the possible unidentified risk of congenital leukemia.

Neonatal Lymphoma

Neonatal lymphoma is an important blood cancer in the neonate. It has a strong relation to Down syndrome. Cancers are in excess in this condition because of the 20-fold excess of leukemias, whereas malignant solid tumors seem to be globally underrepresented as compared with those in the general population [14]. However, among these tumors, some tumors are in excess: lymphomas, gonadal and extragonadal germ cell tumors, and possibly retinoblastomas and pancreatic and bone tumors [14]. Neoplasms in excess are seen earlier, sometimes in fetal life (leukemias and testicular germ cell tumors) or neonatally (leukemias and lymphoma) and affect mainly male subjects [14]. Because the affected infant usually presents with non-Hodgkin's lymphoma at an early age, it is considered unlikely that an immunoaberration is responsible [15]. Also, a T-cell product including eosinophil differentiation factor is reported as the putative pathophysiologic mechanism [15]. Studies demonstrate an increased prevalence of celiac disease in persons with Down syndrome, leading some organizations and authors to recommend universal screening of children with Down syndrome [16-17]. However, many children with Down syndrome are asymptomatic, and the long-term implications of screening are unknown [16-17]. The complication of celiac disease that leads to mortality in the general population is non-Hodgkin's lymphomas [16-17]. However, the screening for celiac disease is considered not cost effective [16-17]. Dixon et al proposed that although the risk for leukemia was higher in individuals with Down syndrome, these patients had a lower risk of developing solid tumors, with the exception of germ cell tumors, and perhaps retinoblastoma and lymphoma [18]. The exact mechanism by which patients with Down syndrome are predisposed to develop malignancies is unclear [19]. However, presence of the extra chromosome no. 21 is presumed to disrupt the genetic balance which increases generalized susceptibility to genetic and environmental trauma [19]. Furthermore, an increased methotrexate toxicity observed in these patients should also be taken into consideration in designing treatment for Down syndrome children with malignancies [19].

In addition to Down syndrome, lymphoma is also common in the infants with congenital HIV infection [20]. Among patients with congenital immunodeficiencies, non-Hodgkin's lymphomas are the most common tumors of the immune system [20]. Specific forms of HIV-associated Hodgkin's lymphomas are linked to expression of Epstein-Barr virus (EBV)-latent proteins; the newly described DNA virus, Karposi's sarcoma-associated herpesvirus/human herpesvirus-8 (KSHV/HHV-8); and perhaps HIV. Elucidation of the factors that contribute to the high incidence of Hodgkin's lymphoma among patients infected with HIV provides insights into important elements of lymphomagenesis [20]. It is essential that lymphadenopathy be proven infectious and any asymptomatic lymph node enlargement must be considered Hodgkin's disease until proven otherwise [21].

"- Blastoma" Type Malignancy

A. Hepatoblastoma

The prevalence of primary liver cancer varies throughout the world. Hepatoblastoma is the most common pediatric liver malignancy, comprising approximately 1% of all pediatric cancers [22]. The disparate clinical staging systems and histologic classifications that were developed during the last decades, nevertheless, reflect the remaining difficulties and uncertainties in characterizing hepatoblastoma [22]. The exact etiology of this cancer remains undetermine [22]. However, it is noted for the association with Beckwith-Weidemann syndrome, familial adenomatosis polypi, and low birth weight [23]. Hepatoblastoma accounts for approximately 5% of malignancies in childhood [24]. Most HBs fall into epithelial or mixed epithelial and mesenchymal categories [24]. Jia *et al* propose that hepatitis B virus X (HBx) might interfere with the molecular pathway also through binding to and altering the activities of helicases necessary, thereby, increase the mutation rate induced by chemical carcinogens during human liver carcinogenesis. They proposed the association between hepatitis B particle and primary liver cancer [25]. Pongpipat *et al* proposed that hepatitis B infection might be an important risk for development of HB [26]. However, Buckley *et al* said that no evidence was found to support the primary study hypotheses relating to hepatitis infection, maternal estrogen exposure, alcohol consumption, smoking, or potential sources of nitrosamines [27]. Cases of combined hepatitis B infection and hepatoblastoma are sporadically reported [26,28]. Indeed, all human hepatitis B viruses characterized so far express three envelope proteins, pre-S1, pre-S2, and HBs, which are believed to function as binding proteins for the cellular receptor, as targets for immune-mediated virus elimination, and in virion morphogenesis and secretion [26]. The common manifestation of hepatoblastoma is the abdominal mass. Basically, a palpable mass in the abdomen of a child is a serious finding [29]. Hepatoblastoma should always be one of the early differential diagnosis.

B. Neuroblastoma

Neuroblastoma is the second most common solid tumor in children that is metastatic in 70% of patients at the time of diagnosis [30]. The ability of neuroblastoma cells to colonize distant organs like the bone marrow and the bone is the result of close interactions between tumor cells and the microenvironment [30]. Like breast cancer and myeloma, neuroblastoma cells activate osteoclasts to form osteolytic lesions [31]. Activation occurs via the receptor activator of NFkappaB ligand (RANKL) or in the absence of RANKL via activation of bone marrow mesenchymal stem cells and stimulation by these cells of the expression of IL-6, a potent osteoclast activating factor. Several targets for therapeutic intervention can now be identified [31]. PHOX2B is the first bona fide neuroblastoma predisposition gene identified, but is mutated in only a small subset of cases [32]. Somatically acquired alterations at chromosome arms 3p and 11q are highly correlated with acquisition of metastases in the absence of MYCN amplification and may be useful as prognostic markers [32]. Recent reports have described additional complexity in the mechanism of action of transcriptionally active p73 (TAp73) in the induction of cell death [33]. The molecular mechanism through which p73 induces apoptosis involves (i) expression and changes in subcellular localization of scotin, producing an endoplasmic reticulum (ER) stress; and (ii) transactivation of PUMA and Bax, thus determining cell fate [33]. On the contrary, deltaNp73 inhibits apoptosis, thus contributing to the oncogenic potential of neuroblastoma cells [33]. As previously mentioned, neuroblastoma has a high invasion. Considering the bone marrow examination in neuroblastoma, myelofibrosis secondary to metastatic neuroblastoma is a frequent finding [34]. Bone marrow involvement by neuroblastoma is usually associated with the presence of a primary adrenal tumor and occurs only infrequently with extra-adrenal primary origin [34]. Bone marrow involvement is usually present at the time of presentation in case where the primary tumor is located in the adrenal gland [34]. Despite advances in the treatment of neuroblastoma, recurrence and metastases continue to pose major problems in clinical management [35].

For neonate, primary tumours are usually localized retroperitoneally or abdominally [36]. Neuroblastoma is considered as the commonest congenital solid tumor [37]. Luis et al reported that the outcome in the congenital group of neuroblastomas was better that expected, probably because of its abdominal location [37]. On the contrary in dumbbell neuroblastomas, neurological damage at birth seems to be irreversible [37]. Neuroblastoma is characterized by a diversity of clinical behavior ranging from spontaneous remission to rapid tumor progression and death [38]. Neuroblastoma produce catecholamine metabolites which are used as tumour markers [36]. MIBG scintigraphy in addition to ultrasound and nuclear magnetic resonance tomography allow specific imaging of the tumour tissue [36]. Children's Oncology Group recently developed a Neuroblastoma Risk Stratification System that is currently in use for treatment stratification purposes, based on clinical and biologic factors that are strongly predictive of outcome [38]. Basically, the clinical presentation of neuroblastoma is related to primary tumor location, production of metabolically active substances, and the presence of metastatic disease [39]. There are also prognostically important associated syndromes including opsoclonus-myoclonus, Horner's syndrome, neurofibromatosis, and a variety of other neurocristopathies [39]. The histologic features of the tumor are of prognostic significance and are utilized in treatment stratification [39]. Features at diagnosis and those determined by initial operation are combined with biologic prognostic factors to achieve risk group assignment for virtually all patients [39]. Lopez-Aguilar et al reported that the most important prognostic factors were still considered to be age, stage and histology [40].

C. Retinoblastoma

Retinoblastoma is another important pediatric solid tumor. Genetic defects are highly likely in neonatal tumours and include those with a high risk of retinoblastoma [41]. Retinoblastoma is a malignant tumour of the eye ball, which develops as a result of the mutation of both alleles of Rb-1 gene [42]. The retinoblastoma protein, Rb, functions as a tumor suppressor by controlling progression through the cell cycle [43]. Rb function is regulated primarily by its phosphorylation state, which is determined by the complex interaction of multiple kinases and their inhibitors that together form the Rb pathway [43]. Rb protein can also inhibit progression through the cell division cycle, and it physically and/or functionally interacts with important cell cycle regulatory molecules [44]. Cell-specific differences in the effect of Rb loss on genome stability may contribute to the tremendous sensitivity of retinal transition cells to tumorigenesis [45].

Symptoms of retinoblastoma are strabismus, reduced visual acuity and red eye, but the absolutely most important sign is leukokoria (white pupillary reflex) [46]. Important diagnostic tools are ophthalmoscopy, ultrasonography, CT and MRI. The goal of treatment is to destroy all tumour tissue, but not the surrounding tissue [46]. Treatment options are enucleation, chemotherapy, external beam radiation, radioactive isotope plaques, cryotherapy, photocoagulation, or a combination of these depending upon the size and location of the tumor [46-48]. Due to the considerable limitations of the evidence identified, it was not possible to make meaningful and robust conclusions about the relative effectiveness of different treatment approaches for childhood retinoblastoma [47]. The present aim is to avoid primary enucleation and external beam radiation as far as possible [47]. The future may lie in local chemotherapy, hyperthermia, and dynamic phototherapy, accelerated proton beam radiotherapy also has promising prospects [48].

References

[1] Plon SE, Nathanson K. Inherited susceptibility for pediatric cancer. *Cancer J.* 2005 Jul-Aug;11(4):255-67.

[2] Stransky E. Perinatal Leukaemia: a review. *Acta Paediatr Acad Sci Hung* 1967;8:121-44.

[3] Izraeli S. Congenital syndromes and leukemia: clues to pathogenesis. *Rev Clin Exp Hematol* 2003;7:246-60.

[4] Slayton WB, Schibler KR. Congenital bone marrow failure syndromes associated with protean developmental defects and leukemia. *Clin Perinatol* 2000;27:543-58.

[5] Pierce MI. Leukemia in newborn infant. *J Pediatr* 1959; 54: 691 – 706.

[6] Cvetkovic P, Cvetkovic R. Acute leukemia in infant. *Bilt Hematol Trans*fuz 1979;7:119-23.

[7] Kroft SH. Role of flow cytometry in pediatric hematopathology. *Am J Clin Pathol.* 2004 Dec;122 Suppl:S19-32.

[8] Izraeli S. Congenital syndromes and leukemia: clues to pathogenesis. *Rev Clin Exp Hematol.* 2003 Sep;7(3):246-60.

[9] Wattanasirichaigoon S, Supantamart V. Congenital leukemia: a case report. *Med J Ubon Hosp* 1985; 6 : 7-11.

[10] Ketusingh K, Vinchitpun K, Vichitpun C. Congenital leukemia. *J Paediatr Soc Thai* 1962; 1: 15-28.

[11] Suwannasung M. Congenital leukemia: a report of a case of acute myelogenous leukemia. *Chula Med J* 1963; 11 : 18-29.

[12] Resnik KS, Brod BB. Leukemia cutis in congenital leukemia. Analysis and review of the world literature with report of an additional case. *Arch Dermatol* 1993;129:1301-6.

[13] Bresters D, Reus AC, Veerman AJ et al. Congenital leukaemia: the Dutch experience and review of the literature. *Br J Haematol* 2002;117:513-24.

[14] Satge D, Sommelet D, Geneix A, Nishi M, Malet P, Vekemans M. A tumor profile in Down syndrome. *Am J Med Genet.* 1998 Jul 7;78(3):207-16.

[15] Lorenzana AN, Schorin MA. Non-Hodgkin's lymphoma in a neonate with Down's syndrome. Case report and literature review. *Am J Pediatr Hematol Oncol.* 1989 Summer;11(2):186-90.

[16] Swigonski NL, Kuhlenschmidt HL, Bull MJ, Corkins MR, Downs SM. Screening for celiac disease in asymptomatic children with Down syndrome: cost-effectiveness of preventing lymphoma. *Pediatrics.* 2006 Aug;118(2):594-602.

[17] Kawatu D, LeLeiko NS. Screening for celiac disease in asymptomatic children with Down syndrome: cost-effectiveness of preventing lymphoma. *Pediatrics.* 2006 Aug;118(2):816-7.

[18] Dixon N, Kishnani PS, Zimmerman S. Clinical manifestations of hematologic and oncologic disorders in patients with Down syndrome. *Am J Med Genet C Semin Med Genet.* 2006 Aug 15;142(3):149-57.

[19] Kusumakumary P, Vats TS, Ankathil R, Gattamaneni HR, Nair MK. Malignancies in Down syndrome. *Indian J Pediatr.* 1997 Nov-Dec;64(6):873-8.

[20] Aboulafia D. Epidemiology and pathogenesis of AIDS-related lymphomas. *Oncology* (Williston Park). 1998 Jul;12(7):1068-81.

[21] Filston HC. Common lumps and bumps of the head and neck in infants and children. *Pediatr Ann.* 1989 Mar;18(3):180-2, 184, 186.

[22] Schnater JM, Kohler SE, Lamers WH, von Schweinitz D, Aronson DC. Where do we stand with hepatoblastoma? *A review. Cancer.* 2003 Aug 15;98(4):668-78.

[23] Herzog CE, Andrassy RJ, Eftekhari F. Childhood cancers: hepatoblastoma. *Oncologist* 2000;5:445-53.

[24] Wittekind C. Pathology of liver tumors. *Zentralbl Chir* 2000;125:587-91

[25] Jia L, Wang XW, Harris CC. Hepatitis B virus X protein inhibits nucleotide excision repair. *Int J Cancer* 1999; 80:875-9.

[26] Pongpipat D, Suvatte V, Assateerawatts A. Hepatitis B surface antigen and alpha-foetoprotein in paediatric hepatocellular carcinoma and hepatoblastoma in Thailand. *Asian Pac J Allergy Immunol* 1983;1:104-6.

[27] Buckley JD, Sather H, Ruccione K, Rogers PC, Haas JE, Henderson BE, Hammond GD. A case-control study of risk factors for hepatoblastoma. A report from the Childrens Cancer Study Group. *Cancer* 1989;64:1169-7.

[28] Inagaki M, Yagi T, Urushihara N, Shima Y, Sadamori H, Takakura N, Tanaka N, Oda M. Successfully resected hepatoblastoma in a young adult with chronic hepatitis B: report of a case. *Eur J Gastroenterol Hepatol* 2001;13:981-4.

[29] Golden CB, Feusner JH. Malignant abdominal masses in children: quick guide to evaluation and diagnosis. *Pediatr Clin North Am.* 2002 Dec;49(6):1369-92, viii.

[30] Ara T, DeClerck YA. Mechanisms of invasion and metastasis in human neuroblastoma. *Cancer Metastasis Rev.* 2006 Dec;25(4):645-57.

[31] Sohara Y, Shimada H, DeClerck YA. Mechanisms of bone invasion and metastasis in human neuroblastoma. *Cancer Lett.* 2005 Oct 18;228(1-2):203-9.

[32] Maris JM. The biologic basis for neuroblastoma heterogeneity and risk stratification. *Curr Opin Pediatr.* 2005 Feb;17(1):7-13.

[33] Rossi M, Sayan AE, Terrinoni A, Melino G, Knight RA. Mechanism of induction of apoptosis by p73 and its relevance to neuroblastoma biology. *Ann N Y Acad Sci.* 2004 Dec;1028:143-9.

[34] Mills AE, Bird AR. Bone marrow changes in neuroblastoma. *Pediatr Pathol.* 1986;5(2):225-34.

[35] Burchill SA. Micrometastases in neuroblastoma: are they clinically important? *J Clin Pathol.* 2004 Jan;57(1):14-20.

[36] Simon T. Neuroblastoma. *Urologe A.* 2005 May;44(5):543-54; 555.

[37] Albert A, Cruz O, Montaner A, Vela A, Badosa J, Castanon M, Morales L. Congenital solid tumors. A thirteen-year review. *Cir Pediatr.* 2004 Jul;17(3):133-6.

[38] Luis AL, Martinez L, Hernandez F, Sastre A, Garcia P, Queizan A, Tovar JA. Congenital neuroblastomas. *Cir Pediatr.* 2004 Apr;17(2):89-92.

[39] Weinstein JL, Katzenstein HM, Cohn SL. Advances in the diagnosis and treatment of neuroblastoma. *Oncologist.* 2003;8(3):278-92.

[40] Haase GM, Perez C, Atkinson JB. Current aspects of biology, risk assessment, and treatment of neuroblastoma. *Semin Surg Oncol.* 1999 Mar;16(2):91-104.

[41] Lopez-Aguilar E, Cerecedo-Diaz F, Rivera-Marquez H, Valdez-Sanchez M, Sepulveda-Vildosola AC, Delgado Huerta S, Vera-Hermosillo H, Vazquez-Langle JR, Wanzke del Angel V. Neuroblastoma: prognostic factors and survival. Experience in Hospital de Pediatria del Centro Medico Nacional del Siglo XXI and review of the literature. *Gac Med Mex*. 2003 May-Jun;139(3):209-14.

[42] Moore SW, Satge D, Sasco AJ, Zimmermann A, Plaschkes J. The epidemiology of neonatal tumours. Report of an international working group. *Pediatr Surg Int*. 2003 Sep;19(7):509-19.

[43] Kostyk E, Pietrzyk JJ. Genetic background of retinoblastoma. *Med Wieku Rozwoj*. 1999 Jan-Mar;3(1):33-40

[44] Brantley MA Jr, Harbour JW. The molecular biology of retinoblastoma. *Ocul Immunol Inflamm*. 2001 Mar;9(1):1-8.

[45] Goodrich DW, Lee WH. Molecular characterization of the retinoblastoma susceptibility gene. *Biochim Biophys Acta*. 1993 May 25;1155(1):43-61.

[46] Bremner R, Chen D, Pacal M, Livne-Bar I, Agochiya M. The RB protein family in retinal development and retinoblastoma: new insights from new mouse models. *Dev Neurosci*. 2004;26(5-6):417-34.

[47] Kinge B, Tranheim RS, Eide NA. Retinoblastoma--hereditary eye cancer in children. *Tidsskr Nor Laegeforen*. 2004 Jan 22;124(2):183-5.

[48] McDaid C, Hartley S, Bagnall AM, Ritchie G, Light K, Riemsma R. Systematic review of effectiveness of different treatments for childhood retinoblastoma. *Health Technol Assess*. 2005 Dec;9(48):iii, ix-x, 1-145.

[49] Balmer A, Munier F, Zografos L. New strategies in the management of retinoblastoma. *J Fr Ophtalmol*. 2002 Feb;25(2):187-93.

Chapter 5

NEONATAL VITAMIN K DEFICIENCY

INTRODUCTION

Vitamin K (phylloquinone, K1; menaquinone, K2) is a lipid soluble vitamin. It is important for the normal hemostatic process in human beings. Vitamin K is an essential co-factor for the synthesis of several coagulation factor. It is well-known that vitamin K has a strong blood coagulation activity by acting a cofactor for gamma-carboxylase which catalizes the conversion of specific glutamic acid residue to gamma-carboxyglutamic acid residue (Gla) [1]. The vitamin K-dependent (VKD) carboxylase uses the oxygenation of vitamin K to convert glutamyl residues (Glus) to carboxylated Glus (Glas) in VKD proteins, rendering them active in a broad range of physiologies that include hemostasis, apoptosis, bone development, arterial calcification, signal transduction, and growth control [2]. The carboxylase has a high-affinity site that selectively binds VKD proteins, usually through their propeptide, and also has a second low-affinity site of VKD protein interaction [2]. Some of the Gla-containing proteins, such as osteocalcin and matrix Gla protein have been found in calcifying tissues [1]. These proteins are considered to play an important role in Ca-deposition [1]. Recently, vitamin K has emerged as a potential protector against osteoporosis and hepatocarcinoma. Accumulated evidence indicates that subclinical non-hemostatic vitamin K deficiency in extrahepatic tissues, particularly in bone, exists widely in the otherwise healthy adult population. Both vitamin K(1) and K(2) have been shown to exert protective effects against osteoporosis [3]. Vitamin K2 is involved in the gamma-carboxylation of coagulation factors and bone proteins, but it can also bind and activate the steroid and xenobiotic receptor in order to mediate transcription in bone tissue, and has been used to treat osteoporosis [4]. It is also found that Vitamin K2 exerts a more powerful influence on bone than vitamin K1 [5].

Vitamin K usually receives less dietary attention and fewer assays in foods than other fat-soluble vitamins [6]. It is widely distributed in foods, usually at low concentrations [6]. Intestinal bacteria synthesize vitamin K, which presumably helps provide the metabolic requirements for vitamin K [6]. Vitamin K in foods includes phylloquinone (K1) found in plants and several menaquinones (K2) found in animals and synthesized by microorganisms [6]. Booth et al studied the food sources and dietary intakes of vitamin K-1 (phylloquinone) in the American diet and found that the 25- to 30-year-old women and men consumed less than the current Recommended Dietary Allowance (RDA) for vitamin K while formula-fed infants had estimated vitamin K-1 intakes six times greater than the RDA [7]. According to this study, the top contributors to total vitamin K-1 intake were dark-green vegetables, although the fats and oils added to mixed dishes and desserts were also important contributors [7]. The proportion of vitamin K-1 obtained from vegetables increased with age [7]. However, the intake of vitamin K in the pediatric population in the developing countries is usually under RDA. Vitamin K deficiency remains a world-wide problem in the newborn. Vitamin K traverses the placenta from mother to infant very poorly and is present only in very low concentrations in human milk [8]. The hematological disorder due to vitamin K deficiency is still important public health threat all over the world [9].

Vitamin K Deficiency

Vitamin K is a trace element. The human requirement is small but it is required. For more than 60 years, vitamin K-dependent proteins have been known to play an important role in regulating blood coagulation. The current daily recommended dietary allowance for vitamin K is 1 microg/kg [10 - 11]. Advances in analytic techniques and more sensitive clotting factor assays will make it possible to define the human requirement for this vitamin more accurately [11]. Reliable measurements of vitamin K content in foods are now available, and data from several studies of vitamin K intake indicate that the mean intake of young adults is approximately 80 microg phylloquinone/d and that older adults consume approximately 150 microg/day [10]. A substantial part of the population is mildly deficient in vitamin K, and at later ages this deficiency may contribute to increased bone fracture risk, arterial calcification, and cardiovascular disease [9].

A. Effect on Coagulation System

Vitamin K functions as an essential cofactor for the synthesis of the coagulation protein factors II, VII, IX, X and protein C and S by promoting a unique post-translational modification of specific glutamic acid residues to gamma-carboxylglutamic acid, thus mediating calcium binding to phospholipid surfaces [10]. Vitamin K deficiency results in a depletion of liver stores of phylloquinone, decreased plasma levels of vitamin K1, increased levels of K1 epoxide, appearance of noncarboxylated protein (PIVKA), decreased levels of functioning vitamin K-dependent clotting factors and prolongation of the APTT, PT and thrombotest [10]. When the progression of deficiency leads to abnormal clotting tests a generalized bleeding tendency occurs [10]. Many of the features of common chronic disorders, especially connective tissue disorders, are identical to the symptoms of vitamin K deficiencies [10]. The bleeding due to the vitamin K deficiency in newborn in the main problem in hematology [10].

Most of the cases of vitamin K deficiencies are due to the oral anticoagulant therapy. However, there are some conditions that vitamin K deficiency is due to the illness.

Coagulopathies are also common in the critically ill, and are often due to vitamin K deficiency or disseminated intravascular coagulation (DIC) [11]. Acquired bleeding disorders in the developing world also include late vitamin K deficiency bleeding (VKDB) in infants [12]. In this chapter, the neonatal hematological disorder will be focused.

B. Effect on Skeletal System

As previously mentioned, the vitamin K also has significant effect on skeletal system. Recommendations for dietary vitamin K intake have been made on the basis of the hepatic requirements for the synthesis of blood coagulation factors [13]. Accumulating evidence suggests that the requirements for other functions than blood coagulation may be higher [13]. It is believed that vitamin D deficiency is responsible for rickets in infants and osteomalacia in adults, and chronic vitamin D insufficiency induces hyperparathyroidism and reduces bone mineral density, resulting in an increased risk of osteoporosis [14]. However, the additional roles of vitamin K deficiency is widely mentioned. Circulating levels of undercarboxylated osteocalcin may be a sensitive marker of vitamin K inadequacy and have been reported to be increased in both postmenopausal women and individuals who sustained hip fracture [15]. It is also possible that vitamin K indirectly affects the skeleton via control of renal calcium excretion [15]. Osteoclastic function is also inhibited by vitamin K [16]. Recent interesting data from an observational study of healthy young girls (aged 3-16 years) in the United States suggests that better vitamin K status is associated with lower levels of markers of bone resorption and bone formation, suggesting a lower rate of bone turnover [17]. Evidence suggests that dietary phylloquinone intake of <100 microg daily might not be optimal for bone health [18]. Low intake of vitamin K could contribute to osteoporosis and subsequent fracture due to the undercarboxylation of osteocalcin [18]. There is a need for randomized phylloquinone supplementation trials to better understand the role of vitamin K on bone acquisition in growing children [17].

BREAST MILK AND VITAMIN K

Breast milk is the best milk because of anti-infective properties which are unavailable from other foodstuffs. Many studies have suggested that breast-fed infants have lower morbidity and mortality than other infants [19]. The anti-infective properties in breast milk can control bacterial, viral and fungal infections [19]. The two most significant influences on bacterial infection are the maternal immune factors, including milk cells and those factors responsible for acidification of the infant gut and establishment of a vigorous lactobacillus flora [19]. Immunoglobulin is probably the most important of antiviral defense factors in breast milk [19]. Breast milk provides the balanced nutritional requirements to meet the needs of infants and also plays a vital role in the prevention of infection [20]. The separate milk components include lipids, protein, carbohydrates, water, salt, calcium and phosphorus, iron, zinc, copper, manganese, selenium, iodine, fluoride, vitamins D, K, A, E, C, thiamine, riboflavin, niacin, pantothenic acid, pyridoxine, biotin, folate, and cyanocobalamine [21 –

22]. Besides a balanced nutrient composition and a number of conditionally essential nutrients, human milk provides different types and classes of bioactive factors, such as enzymes, hormones, and growth factors, many of which appear to have a role in supporting infantile growth and development [21 - 22].

The breastfed infant has limited sources of vitamin K, as it is transmitted poorly across the placenta and is present in very low concentrations in human milk [23]. Sakurai et al as well as Yamawaki et al proposed that indicate that it was necessary to evaluate individual differences in human milk in order to perform valid research regarding infant formula [24 - 25]. Kojima et al performed a research to determine the concentration of vitamin K including K1 and K2 (MK-n) in the maternal milk of Japanese women [26]. According to this work, K1 and MK-4 were found to be predominant in the milk samples, and the concentration of MK-4 in colostrum was higher than that of MK-4 in mature milk [26]. Kojima et al concluded that the different features of vitamin K1 and MK-7 concentrations in the milk of Japanese women may be due to differences in dietary foods [26].

Comparison of fore and hind milk from the mothers revealed higher vitamin K1 concentrations in hindmilks, suggesting that the lipid content influences the vitamin K1 concentration in maternal milk [27]. For colostral milk there was a significant correlation of vitamin K1 to cholesterol but not to total lipid or phospholipid suggesting a role for cholesterol in the secretion of vitamin K1 into colostral milk [27]. For mature milk correlation coefficients of vitamin K1 with all lipids were low suggesting that at later stages of lactation dietary fluctuations of vitamin K1 may be a more important determinant of the vitamin K1 content of breast milk than the lipid composition [27]. There is limited information available on the vitamin K intake of lactating mothers, concentration of vitamin K1 in breast milk, and the effect of long-term vitamin K1 supplementation of lactating mothers on the vitamin K1 concentration in breast milk. Pietschnig et al reported no influence of maternal dietary intake on vitamin K level in breast milk [28]. However, Greer et al found that in exclusively breastfed infants who receive intramuscular phylloquinone at birth, the vitamin K status as measured by plasma phylloquinone and des-gamma-carboxy-prothrombin concentrations is improved by maternal oral supplements of 5 mg/d phylloquinone through the first 12 weeks of life [29]. The similar finding was also reported by Bolisetty et al in the preterm infants with maternal vitamin K supplementation [30].

Neonatal Vitamin K Deficiency

Neonatal vitamin K deficiency is an important pediatric nutrition disorder. Late hemorrhagic disease of newborn (LHDN) is the most common disorder as a result of neonatal vitamin K deficiency [31]. Basically, LHDN is a manifestation of an underlying disorder or idiopatically from the 8th day to 12 weeks after birth [31 – 33]. The common presenting symptoms are seizures, vomiting, poor feeding and altered sensorium [31]. Intracranial bleed, commonest site being intracerebral and multiple intracranial hemorrhage, is the predominant manifestation [31 - 32]. Visible external bleeding was noted in 1/3rd of patients only [32].

Since LHDN leads to significant morbidity and mortality, it should be prevented by providing vitamin K prophylaxis to all newborns [31]. Vitamin K prophylaxis in the neonate is well accepted and routinely practiced in developed countries. It has not been applied routinely in most developing countries because of problems regarding parenteral administration. The routine dosage of vitamin K prophylaxis 1 mg im or at least 2 mg orally to all neonates is strongly recommended and should be emphasized particularly in developing countries.

As previously described, the vitamin is low in breastmilk and the newborn receiving breastmilk without vitamin K supplementation is prone to develop bleeding. The disorder known as acquired prothrombin complex deficiency or APCD can still be observed in the developing countries [34]. APCD syndrome is an acquired bleeding disorder commonly found in infants [35 – 37]. Vitamin K deficiency has been proved to be the responsible cause [37]. To give the reader some ideas on APCD syndrome in developing countries, some reports on a developing country, Thailand is hereby presented. The incidence of APCD syndrome in Thailand is 1:1400 or 72:100,000 of livebirths [37]. In summary, the characteristic features are intracerebral bleeding, anemia, and mild hepatomegaly occurred mostly in breast fed infants who did not receive vitamin K prophylaxis-at birth [38]. The laboratory findings are low Hct, normal platelet count, prolonged VCT, PTT, PT and positive for PIVKA II [38]. Chittanaswad retrospective study of 23 cases of APCD Syndrome and noted that most of the patients were breastfed. In this series, the common manifestations were intracranial bleeding, pallor, seizure and hepatomegaly [35]. The high mortality due to intracranial bleeding was noted [35]. Similar study by Joncharoenkamol also indicated the high mortality due to intracranial bleeind [36]. For estimation, the mortality rate is 30 per cent and permanent neurological handicap occurs in 30-70 per cent of the survived cases [35 – 37]. Pansatiankul et al noted that the trend of the rate of vitamin K given to infants born in the hospital-based in Bangkok were increased form 51.12 % to 80.35 % and in provincial area from 12.51 % to 35.96 % from 1982 to 1986 in parallel to the increment of the incidence of APCD [38].

Vitamin K Deficiency Bleeding in Infancy

Vitamin K deficiency bleeding (VKDB) as neonatal bleeding is often and may occur after the 4-week neonatal period. The incidence of intracranial VKDB can be reduced by early recognition of the signs of predisposing conditions (prolonged jaundice, failure to thrive) and by prompt investigation of "warning bleeds" [39]. VKDB can be classified by age of onset into early (<24 h), classical (days 1-7) and late (>1 week <6 months), and by etiology into idiopathic and secondary [39]. In secondary VKDB, in addition to breast feeding, other predisposing factors are apparent, such as poor intake or absorption of vitamin K [39].

A. Bleeding in Central Nervous System

As previously mentioned, bleeding in central nervous system is a serious and common manifestation of neonatal deficiency. Diagnostic steps have to be initiated immediately [40]. Infants presenting with spontaneous intracranial hemorrhage due to a significant (inherited) coagulopathy are usually easy to differentiate from non-accidental shaking injury; their bleeding pattern within the brain seems different from non-accidental shaking injury and neurodevelopment outcome appears better [41]. VKDB occurs preferentially (90%) in fully breastfed infants, males are affected nearly twice as often as females [41]. According to the study of Sutor et al, patients who suffered VKDB despite having received vitamin K prophylaxis were older at onset and had less intracranial bleedingthan patients who received none [42]. Extensive subdural hematoma with brain edema and brain death are severe sequele of late manifestation of vitamin K deficiency [43] Mental retard is also another important sequele of intracranial hemorrhage due to vitamin K deficiency [44].

Concerning the laboratory investigation, the Quick value is often pathologically low [42]. Vitamin K dependent factors are low and PIVKA is detectable, whereas vitamin K independent hemostatic parameters are normal or even elevated [42]. The combination of low Quick value and normal fibrinogen as well as platelet level is a good diagnostic indicator which can be confirmed by administration of vitamin K, after which the Quick value will rise within 30 minutes [42]. However, the imaging is the best method to reach the structural diagnosis [45 – 46]. MRI might give a better details than CT scan [46]. Sometimes, CT scan can show intracerebral hematomas with niveau, which are surrounded by high-density rings [47]. Under the states in which blood can separate easily with advance of erythrocyte sedimentation rate, blood clot will adhere to the wall of the hematomas [47]. There might be little deviation in spite of the big hematomas which may be according to the fact that the brain of infancy is incomplete in myelination and contains much water, and that the possibility of bleeding due to vitamin K occurs slowly [47]. In the full-term neonates, there is a high incidence of intraventricular hemorrhage and hemorrhage around the falx [45]. Subdural hemorrhage (SDH) can be seen more frequently and intraventricular hemorrhage less frequently in infants than in full-term neonates [45]. The cases with SDH frequently usually shows accompanying cerebral infarction followed by porencephaly, therefore, SDH with cerebral low density on CT may predict a poor prognosis [45].

In contrast to LHDN, vitamin K deficiency bleeding within the first 24 h of life is caused in most cases by maternal drug intake including coumarins, anticonvulsants, tuberculostatics, during pregnancy [48]. Administration of warfarin is also followed by an increased risk both of fetal intraventricular hemorrhage, and of cerebral microbleedings, which may result in microencephaly and mental retardation [49]. Treatment with coumarol derivatives should therefore be avoided during pregnancy, even in pregnant women with artificial heart valves, and replaced by heparin [49]. Hemorrhage in the newborn related to the use of anticonvulsant drugs during pregnancy occurs very early within the first 24 hours, probably due to increased degradation of vitamin K [49]. Transplacental administration of vitamin K has been shown to prevent neonatal hemorrhage induced by maternal anticonvulsant therapy [49]. In the risk pregnancies, antenatal vitamin K prophylaxis and the consideration of a primary Caesarean section in maternal vitamin K deficiency states [48]. However, Prophylactic administration of vitamin K, especially by intramuscular injection, has been reported to be associated with an increased risk of childhood cancer [49].

B. Gastrointestinal Bleeding

According to the study of Kumar et al, the ratio of functional to total prothrombin was significantly lower in infants with diarrhea [50]. However, there was no significant correlation with breast feeding as the only mode of diet, or the prior administration of antibiotics in infants with diarrhea [50]. Recently, Bay et al performed an interesting study to determine the frequency of vitamin K deficiency and to assess its effects on bleeding in patients with acute and intractable diarrhea [51]. According to this work, the duration of diarrhea was significantly longer in infants with gastrointestinal bleeding [51]. Significant improvement in PT and APTT and an increase in coagulation factors were observed after vitamin K had been administered [51]. Bay et al concluded that coagulation parameters could be improved by the administration of vitamin K to children with deranged PT and APTT and diarrheal illness [51].

C. Articular bleeding

Hemarthosis can be a presentation of VKDB. Differential diagnosis between hemarthrosis resulting from vitamin K deficiency and septic arthritis with disseminated intravascular coagulation is a matter of great importance in such patients [52].

References

[1] Koshihara Y. Vitamin K. *Nippon Rinsho*. 1999 Oct;57(10):2247-53.

[2] Berkner KL. The vitamin K-dependent carboxylase. *Annu Rev Nutr*. 2005;25:127-49.

[3] Kaneki M. Protective effects of vitamin K against osteoporosis and its pleiotropic actions. *Clin Calcium*. 2006 Sep;16(9):1526-34.

[4] Bolander FF. Vitamins: not just for enzymes. *Curr Opin Investig Drugs*. 2006 Oct;7(10):912-5.

[5] Plaza SM, Lamson DW. Vitamin K2 in bone metabolism and osteoporosis. *Altern Med Rev*. 2005 Mar;10(1):24-35.

[6] Parrish DB. Determination of vitamin K in foods: a review. *Crit Rev Food Sci Nutr*. 1980;13(4):337-52.

[7] Booth SL, Pennington JA, Sadowski JA. Food sources and dietary intakes of vitamin K-1 (phylloquinone) in the American diet: data from the FDA Total Diet Study. *J Am Diet Assoc*. 1996 Feb;96(2):149-54.

[8] Greer FR. Vitamin K status of lactating mothers and their infants. *Acta Paediatr Suppl*. 1999 Aug;88(430):95-103.

[9] Vermeer C, Schurgers LJ. A comprehensive review of vitamin K and vitamin K antagonists. *Hematol Oncol Clin North Am.* 2000 Apr;14(2):339-53.

[10] Hathaway WE. Vitamin K deficiency. *Southeast Asian J Trop Med Public Health.* 1993;24 Suppl 1:5-9.

[11] Mercer KW, Gail Macik B, Williams ME. Hematologic disorders in critically ill patients. *Semin Respir Crit Care Med.* 2006 Jun;27(3):286-96.

[12] Isarangkura P, Mahasandana C, Chuansumrit A, Angchaisuksiri P. Acquired bleeding disorders: the impact of health problems in the developing world. *Haemophilia.* 2004 Oct;10 Suppl 4:188-95.

[13] Vermeer C, Shearer MJ, Zittermann A, Bolton-Smith C, Szulc P, Hodges S, Walter P, Rambeck W, Stocklin E, Weber P. Beyond deficiency: potential benefits of increased intakes of vitamin K for bone and vascular health. *Eur J Nutr.* 2004 Dec;43(6):325-35.

[14] Okano T. Vitamin D, K and bone mineral density. Clin Calcium. 2005 Sep;15(9):1489-94.

[15] Binkley NC, Suttie JW. Vitamin K nutrition and osteoporosis. *J Nutr.* 1995 Jul;12 5(7):1812-21.

[16] Zofkova I, Kanceva RL. New drugs with positive effects on bones. *Cas Lek Cesk.* 1997 Jul 30; 136(15):459-63.

[17] Cashman KD. Vitamin K status may be an important determinant of childhood bone health. *Nutr Rev.* 2005 Aug; 6 3(8):284-9.

[18] Ryan-Harshman M, Aldoori W. Bone health. New role for vitamin K? *Can Fam Physician.* 2004 Jul; 50:993-7.

[19] Kunjaranussorn P.Breast milk is the best milk R *Thai Army Med J.* 1979; 32(5): 291-297.

[20] The prevalence and duration of breast-feeding: a critical review of available information. Division of Family Health World Health Organization. *World Health Stat Q.* 1982;35:92-116.

[21] Rodriguez-Palmero M, Koletzko B, Kunz C, Jensen R. Nutritional and biochemical properties of human milk: II. Lipids, micronutrients, and bioactive factors. *Clin Perinatol.* 1999 Jun;26(2):335-59.

[22] Nichols EL, Nichols VN. Human milk: nutritional resource. *Prog Clin Biol Res.* 1981;61:109-46.

[23] Greer FR. Vitamin K in human milk--still not enough. *Acta Paediatr.* 2004 Apr;93(4):449-50.

[24] Sakurai T, Furukawa M, Asoh M, Kanno T, Kojima T, Yonekubo A. Fat-soluble and water-soluble vitamin contents of breast milk from Japanese women. *J Nutr Sci Vitaminol (Tokyo).* 2005; 51:239-47.

[25] Yamawaki N, Yamada M, Kan-no T, Kojima T, Kaneko T, Yonekubo A. Macronutrient, mineral and trace element composition of breast milk from Japanese women. *J Trace Elem Med Biol.* 2005; 19(2-3):171-81.

[26] Kojima T, Asoh M, Yamawaki N, Kanno T, Hasegawa H, Yonekubo A. Vitamin K concentrations in the maternal milk of Japanese women. *Acta Paediatr.* 2004 Apr;93(4):457-63.

[27] von Kries R, Shearer M, McCarthy PT, Haug M, Harzer G, Gobel U. Vitamin K1 content of maternal milk: influence of the stage of lactation, lipid composition, and vitamin K1 supplements given to the mother. *Pediatr Res.* 1987 Nov;22(5):513-7.

[28] Pietschnig B, Haschke F, Vanura H, Shearer M, Veitl V, Kellner S, Schuster E. Vitamin K in breast milk: no influence of maternal dietary intake. *Eur J Clin Nutr.* 1993 Mar;47(3):209-15.

[29] Greer FR, Marshall SP, Foley AL, Suttie JW. Improving the vitamin K status of breastfeeding infants with maternal vitamin K supplements. *Pediatrics.* 1997 Jan;99(1):88-92.

[30] Bolisetty S, Gupta JM, Graham GG, Salonikas C, Naidoo D. Vitamin K in preterm breastmilk with maternal supplementation. *Acta Paediatr.* 1998 Sep;87(9):960-2.

[31] D'Souza IE, Rao SD. Late hemorrhagic disease of newborn. *Indian Pediatr.* 2003 Mar;40(3):226-9.

[32] Pooni PA, Singh D, Singh H, Jain BK. Intracranial hemorrhage in late hemorrhagic disease of the newborn. *Indian Pediatr.* 2003 Mar;40(3):243-8.

[33] Zengin E, Sarper N, Turker G, Corapcioglu F, Etus V. Late haemorrhagic disease of the newborn. *Ann Trop Paediatr.* 2006 Sep;26(3):225-31.

[34] Mingvanich S. APCD syndrome and vitamin K prophylaxis. *Saraburi Hosp Med J.* 1988; 13(2): 9-16.

[35] Chittanaswad B. APCD Syndrome at Loei Hospital.6/2 *Reg Med J.* 1993; 1,1: 7-12.

[36] Jongcharoenkamol B. APCD Syndrome. *Maharat Nakhon Ratchasima Hosp Med Bull.*1988; 12(3): 177-183.

[37] Isarangkura P, Chuansumrit A, Hathirat P. Acquired prothrombin complex deficiency (APCD) syndrome and vitamin K prophylaxia as its prevention. *J Pediatr Soc Thai* 1981; 26(4): 145-151.

[38] Pansatiankul BJ, Isranurug S, Thanasophon Y, Sunakorn P, Ungchusak K. Incidence of acquired prothrombin complex deficiency and the status of vitamin K administration in infants in Thailand. *Bull Dept Med Serv* 1988; 14(10): 761-770.

[39] Sutor AH, von Kries R, Cornelissen EA, McNinch AW, Andrew M. Vitamin K deficiency bleeding (VKDB) in infancy. ISTH Pediatric/Perinatal Subcommittee. International Society on Thrombosis and Haemostasis. *Thromb Haemost.* 1999 Mar;81(3):456-61.

[40] Sutor AH, Pancochar H, Niederhoff H, Pollmann H, Hilgenberg F, Palm D, Kunzer W. Vitamin K deficiency hemorrhages in 4 exclusively breast-fed infants 4 to 6 weeks of age. *Dtsch Med Wochenschr.* 1983 Oct 28;108(43):1635-9.

[41] Vorstman EB, Anslow P, Keeling DM, Haythornthwaite G, Bilolikar H, McShane MT. Brain haemorrhage in five infants with coagulopathy. *Arch Dis Child.* 2003 Dec; 88(12):1119-21.

[42] Sutor AH, Dagres N, Niederhoff H.. Late form of vitamin K deficiency bleeding in Germany. *Klin Padiatr.* 1995 May-Jun;207(3):89-97.

[43] Ries M, Tietze HU, Scharf J. Extensive subdural hematoma with brain edema and brain death. Sequela of late manifestation of vitamin K deficiency. *Monatsschr Kinderheilkd.* 1993 Jan;141(1):26-9.

[44] Suzuki H. Neurological symptoms and etiology of severely retarded children. *No To Hattatsu.* 1990 Nov;22(6):539-45.

[45] Nanba E, Eda I, Takashima S, Ohta S, Ohtani K, Takeshita K. Intracranial hemorrhage in the full-term neonate and young infant: correlation of the location and outcome. *Brain Dev.* 1984;6(5):435-43.

[46] Umemura A, Takagi T, Nagai H. A case of intracranial hemorrhage in a young infant due to vitamin K deficiency: comparison of MRI and CT findings. *No To Hattatsu.* 1989 Jul;21(4):385-9.

[47] Nishio T, Nohara R, Aoki S, Sai HS, Izumi H, Miyoshi K, Morikawa Y, Mizuta R. Intracranial hemorrhage in infancy due to vitamin K deficiency: report of a case with multiple intracerebral hematomas with ring-like high density figures. *No To Shinkei.* 1987 Jan;39(1):65-70.

[48] Renzulli P, Tuchschmid P, Eich G, Fanconi S, Schwobel MG. Early vitamin K deficiency bleeding after maternal phenobarbital intake: management of massive intracranial haemorrhage by minimal surgical intervention. *Eur J Pediatr.* 1998 Aug;157(8):663-5.

[49] Astedt B. Antenatal drugs affecting vitamin K status of the fetus and the newborn. *Semin Thromb Hemost.* 1995;21(4):364-70.

[50] Kumar R, Marwaha N, Marwaha RK, Garewal G. Vitamin K deficiency in diarrhoea. *Indian J Pediatr.* 2001 Mar;68(3):235-8.

[51] Bay A, Oner AF, Celebi V, Uner A. Evaluation of vitamin K deficiency in children with acute and intractable diarrhea: *Adv Ther.* 2006 May-Jun;23(3):469-74.

[52] Naveh Y, Berant M, Bialik V. Vitamin K deficiency presenting with hemarthrosis. *J Pediatr Orthop.* 1984 Sep;4(5):630-2.

Chapter 6

Blood Transfusion and Exchange for Neonate

Blood Transfusion for Neonate

Blood transfusion is a general practice in medicine. It is useful for many conditions. The main indication of blood transfusion is for life saving. There are many types of blood transfusions and those types can be applied in neonatology.

A. Whole Blood Transfusion

Whole blood transfusion is rarely indicated in transfusion medicine at present. The transfusion of fresh whole blood (FWB) for trauma-induced coagulopathy is unusual in civilian practice. However, Kauvar et al said that FWB transfusions were most frequent when demands for massive transfusions wiped out existing blood supplies [1]. They noted that FWB patients had the highest blood product requirements but mortality did not differ significantly between FWB and non-FWB patients overall or for massively transfused patients [1]. They propose that FWB might be used in some specific conditions such as during war [1]. Repine et al proposed that the risk: benefit ratio of FWB transfusion favors its use under extreme and austere circumstances [2] FWB may, at times, be advantageous even when conventional component therapy is available [2]. The FWB transfusion is also limited used in neonatology.

B. Fresh Frozen Plasma

The main indication of fresh frozen plasma (FFP) is the replacement of plasma, not cellular component. FFP is heavily used in massive transfusion. Although FFP can partially correct abnormal coagulation, a recent systematic review revealed no randomized trials showing clinical benefit [3]. Although the overall risks of FFP is low, it the least safe blood component, due to immunologic reactions such as allergy/anaphylaxis, transfusion-related acute lung injury (TRALI) and hemolysis due to anti-A or anti-B if transfused across ABO groups [3]. TRALI, an acute syndrome of dyspnoea, hypoxia and pulmonary 'white-out' is now a major cause of transfusion-related death [3]. According to an audit survey in a developing country, the use of FFP for volume support in trauma, massive bleeding and burns, routine requests without identified indication in cardiac bypass surgery, and prophylactic use in the perioperative period can be the basis for recommendations to minimize the inappropriate use of FFP in the future [4].

For neonate, the frequency of specific diseases that might necessitate the administration of FFP differs from that in adults. The plasma levels of many procoagulant factors and important anticoagulants are lower in neonates than in other age groups, however, healthy neonates show no easy bruising, no increased bleeding during surgery, and excellent wound healing [5]. The good primary hemostasis in neonates despite poor in vitro platelet function seems to be due mainly to a very high von Willebrand factor and the presence of more high-multimeric subunits of von Willebrand factor than later in life [5- 6]. Since healthy neonates and young infants have excellent hemostasis, there is absolutely no indication to correct these values to adult's norms prior to invasive procedures by administering FFP [5]. At present, indications for FFP, once used routinely in the support of critically ill infants and children, have become more specific as evolving evidence has confirmed or disproved the efficacy of plasma in various circumstances [6]. FFP is currently indicated to treat the coagulopathies of massive hemorrhage, liver failure and disseminated intravascular coagulation and sepsis [5-6]. Exchange transfusion and extracorporeal membrane oxygenation is additional specific indication for neonates [5]. In congenital clotting factor deficiency, replacement therapy is much more easily administered using a highly specific concentrate [5]. However, when FFP is used to raise the level of the congenitally deficient factor, the huge volume needed to reach sufficiently high plasma levels can frequently be a major problem, therefore, FFP as a replacement therapy in congenital factor deficiency is only indicated when no specific concentrate is available [5].

C. Red Blood Cell Transfusion

Red blood cell transfusion is indicated in cases that need red blood cell such as anemia. Pack red cell (PRC) is the well-known component for red blood cell transfusion. Hematological features indicate that a newborn has a blood volume of 85-125 ml/kg, the foetal haemoglobin is 60-85% and average Hb in full term infant is 18 gm/dl [7]. It severe neonatal anemia is judged, PRC transfusion should be concerned.

Neonatal anemia is an important indication of PRC transfusion. Anemia due to hemorrhage is the most common indication. Hemorrhage can be ante or intra or post natal and it could be external or internal [8]. It could be acute or chronic [8]. Management of acute severe hemorrhage includes packed cell transfusion [8]. However, the red cells transfusions are generally top up exchange transfusions, partial exchange transfusions [7]. Top up- are for investigational losses and correction of mild degrees of anemias, upto to 5-15 ml/kg [7]. They comprise 90% of all neonatal transfusions and are used in low birth babies in special care units for a maximum of 9-10 episodes [7].

There are also some concerns on the adverse effect of repeated RBC transfusion on neonate. The first concern is about the iron overload. Dani et al said that gestational age, blood transfusion volume and iron load by transfusions are associated with the risk of occurrence of ROP in infants with a birthweight of less than 1250 grams [9]. Dani et al also found that plasma non-transferrin bound iron is significantly increased in preterm infants for three hours after PRC transfusion, but this is not associated with significant changes in oxidative stress [10]. Another important concern is the effect on immune system. HLA alloimmunization can be expected. The leukocyte filter technique has been shown to be effective in preventing HLA alloimmunization and transfusion reactions but the price is rather high [11-12]. For the inverted centrifugation technique, only transfusion reactions were effectively prevented and the HLA alloimmunization continued to develop [11].

D. White Blood Cell Transfusion

White blood cell transfusion is not indicated at present due to the high prevalence of blood borne transfusion. The replacement of white blood cell which is the old indication of buffy coat administration is now replaced by the administration of granulocyte stimulating factor. However, there are some practices of granulocyte transfusions in the cases with severe neonatal sepsis [13-15]. According to a recent Cochrane review, there is inconclusive evidence from randomized control trials to support or refute the routine use of granulocyte transfusions in neonates with sepsis and neutropaenia to reduce mortality and morbidity [13]. Researchers can be encouraged to conduct adequately powered multicentre trials of granulocyte transfusions to clarify their role in neonates with sepsis and neutropaenia [13].

E. Platelet Transfusion

Platelet is a part of cell circulating in the blood stream. Platelet, white blood cell (granulocyte) and red blood cell (erythrocyte) are the three important cellular components of blood. For production of platelet, bone marrow is the factory site. Within the bone marrow, megakaryocytopoiesis involves the commitment of haematopoietic stem cells, and the proliferation, maturation and terminal differentiation of the megakaryocytic progenitors [16]. The main function of platelet is in hemostasis process. Concerning the normal hemostasis process, after the episode of hemorrhage, the vasoconstriction is the first response. Coagulation due to coagulation factors to derive fibrin to weave at the wound occurs and the platelet in the blood stream will be entrapped at that site and result in the wound healing. This process must be balanced by the fibrinolysis system to derive homeostasis. Hence, it can be said that platelet is necessary for human beings and defects of platelet, in function or amount, can result in hematological abnormality. Platelet transfusion is a type of blood transfusion. A platelet transfusion is given in the same manner as whole blood. At present, platelet transfusion is widely used in transfusion medicine. There are two important indications for platelet transfusion at present, prophylaxis and therapy. The most important indication for platelet transfusion is the treatment of bleeding episodes in thrombocytopenic patients due to bone marrow aplasia, leukaemia, or chemotherapy of various malignancies [17]. ABO and HLA typing are carried out on donors and recipients [17]. Due to the high polymorphism of the HLA system, it is, however, difficult to find a compatible donor-recipient pair [17]. The indications of important platelet products are presented in Table 2. While many advances have been made in platelet transfusion technology, problems remain [18]. These include the short storage life of liquid-stored platelets and the frequent development of alloantibodies (the refractory state) in patients receiving a number of transfusions [18].

Similar to other blood components transfusion, complications due to platelet transfusion is documented. Refractoriness is the most important complication of platelet transfusion therapy, occurring in about 50% of patients receiving repeated transfusions [19]. Lack of adequate post-transfusion platelet count increments - platelet refractoriness - is a complication of chronic platelet support shown by 5-15% of chronic platelet recipients [20]. Basically, refractoriness is usually defined as the occurrence of 2-3 post-transfusion platelet count increments, corrected for the patient's size and number of administered platelets, at 10-60 minutes and at 18-24 hours post-transfusion below 4,500-5,000 and 2,500 platelets per microliter respectively [20]. Generally, refractoriness is associated with clinical and pharmacological causes in most cases, however, in those cases in which refractoriness is due to immune factors, anti-HLA antibodies are most frequently implicated [20]. The major causes are HLA alloimmunization and non-immune platelet consumption associated with clinical factors such as septicaemia, DIC and splenomegaly [19]. Initial management of alloimmunized patients who are refractory to platelet transfusions from random donors is the use of HLA-matched platelet transfusions, which improve responses to transfusions in about 65% of patients [19].

In neonate, the platelet transfusion is also indicated for the cases with severe thrombocytopenia. Basically, thrombocytopenia occurs in up to a third of preterm neonates admitted to intensive care units [21]. In these babies, thrombocytopenia typically presents in one of two patterns: early-onset thrombocytopenia occurring within 72 hours of birth and late-onset thrombocytopenia which develops after 72 hours [21]. More details on neonatal thrombocytopenia can be found in another chapter in this book. It is noted that late-onset neonatal thrombocytopenia is usually due to bacterial sepsis or necrotising enterocolitis (NEC); it is often severe (platelets <50 x 10(9)/l), prolonged and requires treatment with platelet transfusions [21]. There is a new concern on platelet transfusion in neonate with NEC. It should be noted that platelet transfusions contain a variety of bioactive factors, including platelet activating factor (PAF), which can augment systemic inflammatory processes [22]. A growing body of evidence that incriminates PAF in the pathogenesis of NEC has emerged over the past few decades from both animal and human data [22]. Both severe thrombocytopenia and multiple platelet transfusions have been associated with increased mortality, but it is admittedly difficult to differentiate between the effects of the underlying disease and the effects, if any, of the platelet transfusions [22].

F. Coagulation Factor Transfusion

Coagulation factor transfusion is an important tool for treatment of the patients with Hemophilia [23-24]. The clotting factor can be prepared from the donated blood. The problem on finding of blood donor and donor selection should be mentioned. In addition, the problem of blood borne infection in the present day should be stated. Human immunodeficiency virus (HIV), hepatitis B virus (HBV) and hepatitis C virus (HCV) in the blood supply are the important problematic blood borne transmitted diseases. In general, cryoprecipitate transfusion is the widely used coagulation factor transfusion for the cases with hemophilia [23-25]. According to the study of Evatt et al, over a lifetime of treatment (60 years), the cumulative risk of HIV exposure for a person with haemophilia receiving monthly infusion of cryoprecipitate prepared from plasma is significant, 2% in the USA and 40% in Venezuela [24]. Considering the cumulative risk for transmitting HIV to patients with haemophilia through cryoprecipitate treatment, medical care providers should carefully evaluate the use of cryoprecipitate in any but emergency conditions or when no virally inactivated products are available [24]. In more affluent countries, the debate in recent years has focused on the relative merits of plasma versus recombinant products [23]. Coagulation factor concentrates are expensive, and cost-benefit and quality-of-life studies will assume an increasing importance in guiding the selection of products [23]. Looking to the future, genetic engineering offers the potential to create coagulation factors with enhanced properties, such as reduced immunogenicity and prolonged half-life [23].

Blood Exchange for Neonate

Blood exchange is widely practiced in neonatology. There are two main types of blood exchange, total blood exchange transfusion and partial blood exchange transfusion.

Partial exchange transfusion is traditionally used as the method to lower the Hct and treat hyperviscosity; however, it is unclear whether this is an effective approach in preventing the long-term neurologic consequences [26]. Partial exchange transfusions are done for symptomatic anemia, where Hb<10 g/dl, it is indicated in polycythemia and hyperviscosity syndromes. Exchange volume = Blood volume x (observed Hct-Desired HCt) divided observed Hct. More details on the treatment of polycythemia by partial blood exchange can be seen in another chapter on polycythemia in this book. Total blood exchange is mainly indicated for the neonate with the problem of severe hyperbilirubinemia [27]. The main aim is to prevent the important complication, kernicterus. More details on hyperbililubinemia can also be seen in another chapter in this book. The main concept of blood exchange is to get rid of the unwanted component within the patients' blood and replace with the new satisfied blood. However, there are also other important general indication of total blood exchange such as severe malaria and leptospirosis. Transfusion-acquired malaria in a neonate is uncommon and factors such as drug resistance and concomitant G6PD deficiency can cause treatment difficulties [28]. Therapy by total blood exchange is aiming at correction of anemia, decreasing parasitemia and removal of G6PD-deficient cells to allow successful use of quinine [28]. On the other hand, it should be noted that malaria can also be result of the total blood exchange in the neonate [29]. The risk of transfusion-induced malaria may be increasing in areas endemic for malaria. Careful blood donor selection and blood donor education may minimize this risk [29]. For leptospirosis, there has been no report on the total blood exchange for treatment of leptospirosis in the newborns. This may be due to the fact that the leptospirosis in newborn is very rare.

Blood Donation for Neonate

Blood donation is important for getting of blood and blood product. There is a question if a neonate can be a donor. It is not surprised that cord blood donation is available, however, the donation from the venous blood is very rare. More details on cord blood banking can be seen in another chapter in this book. However, new idea on baby blood donor program is proposed. A good example is the baby blood donor program at Georgia. The concept is to get the CMV-negative blood, which is extremely available from adulthood, to treat newborn. Indeed, CMV might be non serious infection in adulthood but it is very serious for the neonate [30]. According to this program, the blood bank workers will collect 50 pints of CMV-negative blood each day, seven days a week to fulfill the needs of pediatric patients [30]. This blood Donor Program comprised of dependable donors donating every 56 days [30].

Transfusion Practice for Jehovah's Witness Neonates

Due to the principle of Jehovah's Witness, blood and blood product transfusion is not allowable. It is well established from clinical physiology that a hemoglobin concentration lower than 10 g/dl is enough to serve the oxygen demand of the tissues, but transfusion of erythrocytes is still liberally carried out [31]. Data obtained from Jehovah's Witnesses, who categorically refuse blood transfusions, demonstrate that they have an outcome similar to patients who are transfused [31]. The alternative treatment program for Jehovah's Witness is necessary [32-34]. For Jehovah Witness patients the additional responsibilities of surgeon, anesthetist and intensivist represent a particular challenge. A "therapeutic" contract needs to be established at the very outset specifying the commitment and undertaking of each party [32]. Lakatos reported a successful protocol for treatment of an ABO-incompatible term infant girl born to parents who are Jehovah's Witnesses [32] According to Lakatos et al report, alternative treatments of orally administered D-penicillamine (300 mg/kg per day divided in three doses for 3 days), phototherapy, intravenous fluids, and recombinant human erythropoietin (200 U/kg subcutaneously on every second day for 2 weeks). Herein, we report the outcome of this baby, who was discharged from the our unit in good condition after treatment [32]. Kappas et al reported an interesting trial to determine if they could use the potent inhibitor of bilirubin production, Sn-Mesoporphyrin (SnMP) 6 micromol/kg birth weight, single dose), to resolve the troubling medical-legal issues in such situations in 2 infants with hemolytic disease of the newborn who required exchange transfusions for severe hyperbilirubinemia but whose Jehovah's Witness parents rejected the procedure [34]. They got success in their trial [34]. This report confirms the efficacy of SnMP in terminating progression of hyperbilirubinemia in infants in whom phototherapy had failed to sufficiently control the problem and whose parents, for religious reasons, will not permit exchange transfusions [34]. Kappas et al concluded that interdiction of severe hyperbilirubinemia by inhibiting the production of bilirubin with SnMP could be an effective alternative to the use of exchange transfusion in the management of severe newborn jaundice that has not responded sufficiently to light treatment to ease concern about the development of bilirubin encephalopathy [34].

Fetal Transfusion

Fetal transfusion is the new concept of treatment of fetal anemia. The perinatal outcome of the anaemic fetus has dramatically improved over the last 20 years, as a result of early recognition of the problem and treatment by intrauterine transfusion [35]. Prenatal Doppler study is a noninvasive venue in the diagnosis and treatment of fetal anemia [36]. Once the diagnosis of fetal anemia is made, the patient will be asked to undergo an algorithm to investigate the definite cause of anemia, along with simultaneous ultrasound-guided intravascular fetal transfusion in selected cases [36]. Intrauterine transfusion therapy of both red cells and platelets, are being further refined to allow the prompt recognition and treatment of fetal cytopenias [37]. Fetal intraperitoneal transfusion in the treatment of severe red blood cell alloimmunization was first reported by Liley in 1963 [38]. Since then, major advancements have included intravascular techniques and fetal paralysis [38]. According to the study Schumacher and Moise, for pregnant patients presenting with severe red blood cell alloimmunization remote from term, fetal transfusion remains the best available therapeutic option [38]. It is a safe procedure with a perinatal loss rate of approximately 1-3%, and overall neonatal survival exceeds 80% [38]. Fetal transfusion is presently accepted as a rational treatment of the anemic fetus, with improved outcome for all such fetuses and, particularly, for the hydropic, moribund group [39]. Most cases of red cell alloimmunization associated with fetal anemia are caused by the antibody to the D red cell antigen [40]. The intravascular transfusion of red cells to a hydropic fetus in such cases has notably improved survival [40]. Nonimmune hydrops fetalis due to maternal parvovirus infection has also been treated successfully with the intravascular transfusion of red cells, whereas fetomaternal hemorrhage has not proved amenable to such therapy [40]. Concern on the immunomodulation due to intrauterine transfusion is set. Vietor et al reported that after the course of intrauterine transfusion treatment a memory response against donor antigens was generated and this was also reflected by an increase in CD3/CD45RO+ T-cells and modulation of T cell receptor Vbeta (TCRBV) repertoire [41].

References

[1] Kauvar DS, Holcomb JB, Norris GC, Hess JR. Fresh whole blood transfusion: a controversial military practice. *J Trauma.* 2006 Jul;61(1):181-4.

[2] Repine TB, Perkins JG, Kauvar DS, Blackborne L. The use of fresh whole blood in massive transfusion. *J Trauma.* 2006 Jun;60(6 Suppl):S59-69.

[3] MacLennan S, Williamson LM. Risks of fresh frozen plasma and platelets. *J Trauma.* 2006 Jun;60(6 Suppl):S46-50.

[4] Prathiba R, Jayaranee S, Ramesh JC, Lopez CG, Vasanthi N. An audit of fresh frozen plasma usage in a tertiary referral centre in a developing country. *Malays J Pathol.* 2001 Jun;23(1):41-6.

[5] Muntean W. Fresh frozen plasma in the pediatric age group and in congenital coagulation factor deficiency. *Thromb Res.* 2002 Oct 31;107 Suppl 1:S29-32.

[6] Goldenberg NA, Manco-Johnson MJ. Pediatric hemostasis and use of plasma components. *Best Pract Res Clin Haematol.* 2006; 19(1):143-55.

[7] Radhakrishnan KM, Chakravarthi S, Pushkala S, Jayaraju J. Component therapy. *Indian J Pediatr.* 2003 Aug;70(8):661-6.

[8] Lokeshwar MR, Dalal R, Manglani M, Shah N. Anemia in newborn. *Indian J Pediatr.* 1998 Sep-Oct;65(5):651-61.

[9] Dani C, Reali MF, Bertini G, Martelli E, Pezzati M, Rubaltelli FF. The role of blood transfusions and iron intake on retinopathy of prematurity. *Early Hum Dev.* 2001 Apr;62(1):57-63.

[10] Dani C, Martelli E, Bertini G, Pezzati M, Rossetti M, Buonocore G, Paffetti P, Rubaltelli FF. Effect of blood transfusions on oxidative stress in preterm infants. *Arch Dis Child Fetal Neonatal Ed.* 2004 Sep;89(5):F408-11.

[11] Chuansumrit A, Nathalang O, Wangruansathit S, Hathirat P, Chiewsilp P, Isarangkura P. HLA alloimmunization in patients receiving multitransfusions of red blood cells. *Southeast Asian J Trop Med Public Health.* 2001 Jun;32(2):419-24.

[12] Tan KK, Lee WS, Liaw LC, Oh A. A prospective study on the use of leucocyte-filters in reducing blood transfusion reactions in multi-transfused thalassemic children. *Singapore Med J.* 1993 Apr;34(2):109-11.

[13] Mohan P, Brocklehurst P. Granulocyte transfusions for neonates with confirmed or suspected sepsis and neutropaenia. *Cochrane Database Syst Rev.* 2003; (4):CD003956.

[14] Baley JE, Stork EK, Warkentin PI, Shurin SB. Buffy coat transfusions in neutropenic neonates with presumed sepsis: a prospective, randomized trial. *Pediatrics.* 1987 Nov;80(5):712-20.

[15] Wheeler JG, Chauvenet AR, Johnson CA, Block SM, Dillard R, Abramson JS. Buffy coat transfusions in neonates with sepsis and neutrophil storage pool depletion. *Pediatrics.* 1987 Mar;79(3):422-5.

[16] Deutsch VR, Tomer A. Megakaryocyte development and platelet production. *Br J Haematol.* 2006 Jul 20;

[17] Seidl S, Kilp M. The current status of platelet and granulocyte transfusions. *Haematologia (Budap).* 1980; 13(1-4):145-54.

[18] Kelton JG, Blajchman MA. Platelet transfusions. *Can Med Assoc J.* 1979 Nov 17;121(10):1353-8.

[19] Murphy MF, Waters AH. Clinical aspects of platelet transfusions. *Blood Coagul Fibrinolysis.* 1991 Apr;2(2):389-96.

[20] Rubella P. A mini-review on platelet refractoriness. *Haematologica.* 2005 Feb;90(2):247-53.

[21] Chakravorty S, Murray N, Roberts I. Neonatal thrombocytopenia. *Early Hum Dev.* 2005 Jan;81(1):35-41.

[22] Fernandes CJ, O'Donovan DJ. Platelet transfusions in infants with necrotizing enterocolitis. *Curr Hematol Rep.* 2006 Mar;5(1):76-81.

[23] Giangrande PL. Blood products for hemophilia: past, present and future. *BioDrugs.* 2004;18(4):225-34.

[24] Evatt BL, Austin H, Leon G, Ruiz-Saez A, De Bosch N. Haemophilia therapy: assessing the cumulative risk of HIV exposure by cryoprecipitate. *Haemophilia.* 1999 Sep;5(5):295-300.

[25] Srivastava A. Factor replacement for haemophilia--should cryoprecipitate be used? *Haemophilia.* 1999 Sep;5(5):301-5.

[26] Schimmel MS, Bromiker R, Soll RF. Neonatal polycythemia: is partial exchange transfusion justified? *Clin Perinatol.* 2004 Sep;31(3):545-53, ix-x

[27] Schwoebel A, Gennaro S. Normal endothelium. *Handb Exp Pharmacol.* 2006; (176 Pt 1): 1-40.

[28] Virdi VS, Goraya JS, Khadwal A, Seth A. Neonatal transfusion malaria requiring exchange transfusion. *Ann Trop Paediatr.* 2003 Sep;23(3):205-7.

[29] Shulman IA, Saxena S, Nelson JM, Furmanski M. Neonatal exchange transfusions complicated by transfusion-induced malaria. *Pediatrics.* 1984 Mar;73(3):330-2.

[30] Baby Blood Donor Program. Available online at www.parenttoparentofga.org/ Spring0307.htm

[31] von Bormann B. Clinical aspects of packed red cell transfusion: Lessons learned from Jehovah's Witnesses? *Anaesthesist.* 2007 Mar 14;

[32] Chassot PG, Kern C, Ravussin P. Hemorrhage and transfusion: the case of Jehovah's witnesses. *Rev Med Suisse.* 2006 Nov 22;2(88):2674-6, 2678-910.5.

[33] Bausch LC. Blood transfusions and the Jehovah's Witness--neonatal perspectives. *Nebr Med J.* 1991 Aug;76(8):283-4.

[34] Kappas A, Drummond GS, Munson DP, Marshall JR. Sn-Mesoporphyrin interdiction of severe hyperbilirubinemia in Jehovah's Witness newborns as an alternative to exchange transfusion. *Pediatrics.* 2001 Dec;108(6):1374-7.

[35] Harrington K, Fayyad A. Prediction of fetal anaemia. *Curr Opin Obstet Gynecol.* 2002 Apr;14(2):177-85.

[36] Wataganara T, Wiwanichayakul B, Ruengwuttilert P, Sunsaneevithayakul P, Viboonchart S, Wantanasiri C. Noninvasive diagnosis of fetal anemia and fetal intravascular transfusion therapy: experiences at Siriraj Hospital. *J Med Assoc Thai.* 2006 Jul;89(7):1036-43.

[37] Skupski DW, Wolf CF, Bussel JB. Fetal transfusion therapy. *Obstet Gynecol Surv.* 1996 Mar;51(3):181-92

[38] Schumacher B, Moise KJ Jr. Fetal transfusion for red blood cell alloimmunization in pregnancy. *Obstet Gynecol.* 1996 Jul;88(1):137-50.

[39] Ryan G, Morrow RJ. Fetal blood transfusion. *Clin Perinatol.* 1994 Sep;21(3):573-89.

[40] Moise KJ Jr. Intrauterine transfusion with red cells and platelets. *West J Med.* 1993 Sep;159(3):318-24.

[41] Vietor HE. Immunomodulation induced by intrauterine transfusions. *Eur J Obstet Gynecol Reprod Biol.* 1998 May;78(1):33-5.

Chapter 7

HEMOLYTIC DISEASE OF THE NEWBORN

INTRODUCTION TO BLEEDING DIATHESIS

Newborn bleeding is an important problem in pediatrics. The serious unwanted episode is the hemorrhage in the central nervous system. There are several causes of newborn bleeding. Some causes are congenital, the others are acquired. An accurate diagnosis is critically important in order to implement optimal therapy [1]. Over the last century, several investigators have measured plasma concentrations of hemostatic components in newborns and compared the results to adult values [1].

Some influences of age on hemostasis are: (a) the diagnosis of some congenital factor deficiencies, based on plasma levels, can be difficult due to physiologically low values; (b) despite very low levels of many inhibitors of hemostasis, thrombotic complications are rare; (c) the interaction of anti-coagulants and thrombolytic agents is profoundly influenced by the relative immaturity of hemostasis at birth; and (d) in contrast to the risk of thrombosis, healthy infants are at risk for vitamin K deficiency bleeding due to poor transport of vitamin K across the placenta and plasma concentrations of the vitamin K dependent proteins of less than 50% of adults values [1]. These items should be kept in mind when approach to the management of infants with impaired hemostasis [2].

Clinically, bleeding defects have been identified with an heterogeneous group of clinical disease that differs from one another in etiology, pathogenesis, epidemiology and incidence in population [3]. Bleeding diathesis is the common symptom: bleeding tendency may be mild, moderate or severe, localized or generalized, cutaneous or mucosal, superficial or deep [3]. Bleeding disorders may be classified as a) defects in the primary haemostasis, which include quantitative and qualitative abnormalities of platelets and vascular disorders and b) defects in secondary haemostasis, which include intravascular disorders (blood coagulation) [3]. Similar to general rules in medicine, good history taking and clinical examination are essential in diagnosis of bleeding disorders [3]. History of patient should be taken a) to differentiate acquired from congenital disease and to know the track of hereditary transmission (family history); b) to know exactly the disease's start and the mutual relation with former or accompanying disease; c) mutual relation with drugs use [3]. Subsequently a careful physical examination should be done [3].

Basic Laboratory Investigation for Neonatal Bleeding

The initial laboratory work up for screening patients with bleeding disorders should include first step tests to differentiate bleeding disorders for malignancies of bone-marrow; from virus infections carrying screening of major viruses and from liver abnormalities while the second step laboratory examination includes a) platelet count or estimation of platelet number on peripheral blood smear; b) bleeding time to test small vessel integrity and platelet function; c) aPTT, PT, AP to measure clotting activity; d) fibrinogen determination [3]. However, for the pediatric population, some difference protocol should be mentioned. Evaluation of hemolysis the newborn may be complicated owing to the physiologic changes that occur during this time; however, the newborn period is a time when congenital red cell abnormalities may first present and when maternal factors need to be considered [4]. Hemolytic anemia is the common problem for the newborn that all general practitioner should concern.

The two forms of hemolytic anemia in newborn should be mentioned. Non-spherocytic hemolytic anemias are a heterogeneous group of disorders caused by an ineffective normal-type enzyme or, more commonly, by a structurally abnormal and ineffective mutant enzyme [5]. The other, more common, form is spherocytic hemolytic anaemias. These anemias are usually due to the immune destruction process. When the antenatal patient with an irregular antibody is discovered, her partner should be tested for the antigen. If present, the physician can determine the severity of the disease than can be caused by this antibody [6-7]. Hemce, the examination of red cell as well as immunohematology test should added into the general laboratory investigation for bleeding patients.

Hemolytic Disease of the Newborn

Hemolytic disease of the newborn (HDN) is an important problem in neonatal hematology. HDN is resulted from immunopathological process. occurs due to maternal IgG antibodies crossing the placenta thereby producing hemolysis mainly due to Rh, ABO and Kell groups [8].

A. Rh HDN

The RhD protein is expressed only on human red blood cells (RBC), and is one of the most immunogenic of the blood groups [9]. The RH system is one of the most immunogenic and polymorphic human blood group system [10]. It is of clinical importance since the alloantibody (anti-D) can hemolyse D positive RBC after blood transfusion, or cause HDN [9]. Rh (Rhesus) proteins (D, CcEe) are expressed in red cells (RBC) in association with other membrane proteins (RhAG, LW, CD47 and GPB) [10]. By interacting with the spectrin-based skeleton through protein 4.2 and ankyrin, the Rh complex contributes to the maintenance of the mechanical properties of the erythrocyte membrane [10]. The immunogenicity of D is better understood with the knowledge of the genetic basis of the protein(s) involved, the molecular orientation in the RBC membrane, and the nature of the cellular immune response to proteins [9].

When an RhD negative mother is exposed to the RhD positive red cells (usually as transplacental haemorrhage), she develops allo-anti-D which crosses the placenta and then results in the destruction of fetal red cells [11]. Clinical manifestations of RhD HDN range from asymptomatic mild anaemia to hydrops fetalis or stillbirth associated with severe anaemia and jaundice [11]. HDN was a significant cause of fetal mortality and morbidity until the introduction of amniocentesis, intrauterine transfusion, controlled early delivery and exchange transfusion in the management of severely alloimmunised women and their fetuses [11]. A maternal high titer (> or =64) of anti-Di(b) is associated with a higher risk of severe hyperbilirubinemia for mismatched newborns [12]. A systematic approach to the Rh HDN involves an obstetric history of previous isoimmunized baby, timing and regular monitoring of maternal Rh antibodies and pigment assay of amniotic fluid [8]. Timely decision regarding in utero transfusion and early termination of pregnancy based on the maternal monitoring has radically improved the outcome of these babies [8].

Jaundice caused by hemolysis continues to challenge practitioners caring for infants in the NICU [13]. Bilirubin levels can rise quickly in the first days of life, and interventions must be prompt to prevent side effects related to hyperbilirubinemia [13]. Anti-D immune globulin has reduced the incidence of Rh sensitization [14]. Intrauterine transfusions have become routine to treat fetal anemia [14]. Once an affected infant is born, several recent improvements in neonatal care have aided in the treatment of hyperbilirubinemia [14]. These include improved phototherapy, such as fiberoptic delivery systems, and intravenous immunoglobulin [13-14]. Conventional treatments such as hydration and phototherapy are common, but new studies suggest that use of intravenous immunoglobin (IVIG) as an additional treatment may prevent the need for exchange transfusion in some babies [12]. Daglogu et al reported that the number of exchange transfusions needed decreased significantly as a result of IVIG treatment and no side-effects of were seen [15].

Anti-D prophylaxis is the most successful clinical application of antibody-mediated immune suppression [16]. Passive IgG anti-D is given to Rh D-negative women to prevent immunisation to fetal Rh D-positive red blood cells and subsequent haemolytic disease of the newborn [16]. It is hypothesised that although clearance and destruction of the antigenic red blood cell may be a contributing factor in preventing immunisation, down-regulation of antigen-specific B cells through co-ligation of B cell receptors and inhibitory IgG Fc receptors must also occur [16].

B. ABO HDN

ABO is another common HDN but it is not as severe as Rh HDN. ABO hdn is a common cause of neonatal hyperbilirubinemia. The immunologic ABO antibodies and its titration test, especially, elution test are important for prognosis of HDN [17]. It is stated that the direct antiglobulin (Coombs') test (DAT) may be negative in ABO HDN [18]. Thus, significant jaundice in neonates who are A-B incompatible with their mothers but DAT test negative is often attributed to isoimmunization and another diagnosis is not sought [18]. In DAT-negative newborns with significant jaundice or increased bilirubin production, even if ABO-incompatible, a cause other than isoimmunization should be sought [18]. Herschel et al proposed that isoimmunization was unlikely to be the cause of hemolysis in ABO-incompatible but direct antiglobulin test-negative neonates [18]. Due to the low ratio of observed to expected significant clinical events among ABO incompatible mother-infant pairs, and the multiplicity of mechanisms that diminish hemolysis, Waldron and de Alarcon speculated that severe ABO hemolytic disease of the newborn occurred when there was a specific failure in one of these preventive mechanisms [19].

Han et al performed an interesting study to determine whether it was cost effective to screen for ABO incompatability. According to this study, the incidence of HDN due to ABO incompatibility was 3.7% of all group O mothers [20]. Coombs' test, maternal antibody titre, cord bilirubin and haptoglobin levels were of low predictive value for severe HDN due to ABO incompatibility [20]. The data further support the notion that it is not cost effective to screen for ABO incompatibility [20]. Levine and Meyer also found that DAT was neither diagnostic nor predictive of severity [21]. Chen and Ling proposed that ABO incompatible newborn infants with maternal IgG anti-A or anti-B titers > or = 512X, cord bilirubin levels > or = 4 mg/dl or positive direct Coombs' test of the cord blood represented a "high risk" category, and should be placed in hospital where frequent re-evaluation and appropriate therapy are available [22]. Whyte and Graham mentioned that the spin DAGT, despite the weakness of the reaction, reliably identifies infants at risk from severe ABO HDN and is sufficiently sensitive to be used as a single screening test for the early detection of the disorder [23].

Although ABO HDN is usually not severe severe hemolysis occasionally occurs, and some cases require exchange transfusion. The enormous laboratory burden of IgG-anti-A, -B testing during pregnancy is in poor conformity with clinically demonstrable illness [24]. This discrepancy is due to the rarity of true ABO incompatibilities and not to the ineffectiveness of laboratory investigations [24]. The frequency of the haemolytic disease of the newborn due to ABO-incompatibility (ABO-HDN), requiring treatment, is with approximately 5% of all hyperbilirubinemias in newborns lower than usually expected [24]. Toy et al reported that suggested that there were small ethnic differences in the prevalence of positive DAT results in group A infants born to group O mothers, but the prevalence of clinical disease which required exchange transfusion does not differ significantly among Asian, Black, Hispanic and Caucasian infants [25]. The reticulocyte count, a positiveDAT, and the presence of a sibling with neonatal jaundice were determined to be the good predictors for the development of significant hyperbilirubinemia and severe HDN [26]. The ADCC assay with maternal serum is the most sensitive assay to predict ABO-HDN, and the combination of the ADCC assay with A or B antigen density determination the most specific test [27]. A serum bilirubin measurement and the use of the critical bilirubin levels of 4 mg/dL and 6 mg/dL at the sixth hour of life will predict nearly all newborns who will have significant hyperbilirubinemia and those who will develop severe hemolytic disease of the newborn, respectively [26].

Concerning treatment for ABO HDN, a similar protocol to Rh HDN can be applied. However, since the disease is not severe, the phototherpy becomes the most widely used method. Phototherapy is a method to decrease the hyperbilirubinemia, an important consequence of HDN. Rarely, the exchange transfusion is necessary. Similar to RH HDN, the IVIG therapy can reduce the rate of exchange transfusion for treatment of ABO HDN. Although IVIG therapy has been reported in hyperbilirubinemia of Rh hemolytic disease, its use in ABO HDN has been reported in only a few studies [28]. Miqdad et al reported that Administration of IVIG to newborns with significant hyperbilirubinemia due to ABO hemolytic disease with positive direct Coomb's test reduces the need for exchange transfusion without producing immediate adverse effects [28]. Alternative bloodless treatment is also reported for ABO HDN. Alternative treatments of orally administered D-penicillamine (300 mg/kg per day divided in three doses for 3 days), phototherapy, intravenous fluids, and recombinant human erythropoietin (200 U/kg subcutaneously on every second day for 2 weeks) was reported for the success in Jehovah's Witnesses infant [29].

C. Kell HDN

Kell HDN is rare. Basically, the Kell blood group system is complex containing over 20 different antigens [30]. Some of the Kell antigens may be organized in 5 sets of paired alleles with opposing high and low incidence antigens while others are independently expressed [30]. Molecular cloning established that Kell antigens are carried on a 93kDa, type II, membrane glycoprotein [30]. The Kell gene (KEL) is located at 7q 32-36 and spans about 21,5 kb [30- 31]. The coding sequence is organized in 19 exons [30-31]. Sequence analysis of the Kell gene (KEL) established that single base substitutions, resulting in amino acid changes, are responsible for the different phenotypes [31]. Most of the amino acid substitutions, with the exception of the one responsible for expression of KEL6 (Jsa), occur at the amino-terminal half of the protein, a domain that has least amino acid homology with a family of zinc endopeptidases, which include neutral endopeptidase 24.11 and endothelin-converting enzyme-1 [31]. The relative frequency of Kell (K:1) antibodies in pregnant women and a series of cases of Kell hemolytic disease of newborns are sporadic.

Among reproductive-aged women, Kell antibodies are about 60% as frequent as Rho (D) antibodies, but Kell disease is only 3% as common as Rho hemolytic disease [32]. The reason is related to frequent transfusion-alloimmunization by Kell antigen and the low frequency of the K:1 gene among fathers [32]. Kell hemolysis is severe in about half of cases [32]. Amniocentesis is indicated in only a few circumstances: previous child with erythroblastosis fetalis, significant increase in maternal Coombs titer, presence of Kell antigen in the father, and after comparison of the relative risks of hemolytic disease and amniocentesis in each patient [32]. Indeed, determination of fetal red blood cell Kell antigen is possible on fetal red blood cells obtained at 10 weeks of gestation by chorionic biopsy and may contribute to the management of severe Kell-hemolytic disease [32-34].When there is a history of hydrops or the father is Kell-positive and the maternal anti-Kell indirect antiglobulin titer is 8 or greater, amniocentesis should be performed at 16-20 weeks' gestation [33]. Fetal blood sampling followed by fetal intravascular transfusion is indicated if delta OD 450 readings approach the 65% level in modified zone 2 of Liley or if amniocentesis is precluded because of an anterior placenta and there is a history of hydrops or ultrasound evidence of fetal hemolytic disease [33].

Mothers with Kell-positive infants and poor outcome usually have anti-Kell titers greater than or equal to 1:128 at delivery [35]. Mayne et al noted that about 88% of Kell immunized women gave a history of previous transfusion [36]. Spectrophotometric analysis of amniotic fluid (delta optical density at 450 nm) in most cases with poor perinatal outcomes often reveal values of delta optical density at 450 nm in the high midzone of Liley within 1 week of delivery [35]. A policy for management of Kell sensitized pregnancies is outlined, based upon maternal anti-Kell titre and where appropriate fetal blood sampling [35-36].

D. MNS HDN

MNS HDN is first reported by Reid et al in 2000. In this case, the HDN is caused by HDN) caused by anti-Or [37]. The antibody in the mother's serum and in the baby's eluate was identified as anti-Or [37]. At birth, the baby had clinical symptoms of HDN and was transfused with 36 ml of packed RBCs and received phototherapy for eight days [37]. At week 11, the baby's M+N+S+s+Or+ RBCs were negative on the DAT [37].

Non Immune Hemolytic Disorder of the Newborn

As previously mentioned, there are some non immune hemolytic disorders in the newborn. Congenital enzymatic deficiency can be the cause of hemolytic disorder in the newborn. The details on the enzymatic deficiency can be seen in another chapter in this book. The important condition that should be mentioned is the hemolytic uremic syndrome (HUS). This can be the consequence of infection or metabolic disorder in the infant. Indeed, one of the main causes of acute renal failure in the pediatric population. Hemolytic anemia, thrombocytopenia and acute renal failure are the main manifestation of HUS. Concerning the infection, several infections are mentioned for its correlation to HUS in infant. Direct cause-effect relationship between *Bordetella pertussis* infection and HUS was reported in infant [38]. Pneumococcal infection is also frequently mentioned for the correlation to HUS in infant [39-40].

There are also other rare causes of hemolytic disorders in the newborn that should be mentioned. Microangiopathic hemolytic anemia (MAHA) can also be seen in newborn. Congenital MAHA can be seen. Sartori et al reported a case with recurrent MAHA and thrombocytopenia who presented on the first day of life [41]. Remission was maintained only by regular infusions of fresh frozen plasma [41]. Sartori proposed that Congenital MAHA might be a variant of thrombotic thrombocytopenic purpura [41]. Kasabach-Meritt syndrome, a combination of thromobocytopenia, hemolytic anemia, and acute or chronic consumptive coagulopathy in association with rapidly enlarging hemangioma is another rare cause of hemolysis in the newborn [42]. Vincritine is recommended for treatment of this condition. Fatality due to this syndrome can be seen. Retroperitoneal kaposiform hemangioendothelioma is usual common pathological finding in fatal case of Kasabach-Meritt syndrome [43-45].

References

[1] Andrew M. Developmental hemostasis: relevance to hemostatic problems during childhood. *Semin Thromb Hemost.* 1995; 21(4):341-56.

[2] Andrew M. An approach to the management of infants with impaired haemostasis. *Baillieres Clin Haematol.* 1991 Apr;4(2):251-89.

[3] Carnelli V, Dozzi M, Gibelli M, Giovanniello A, Riva F, Seidita C, Stucchi C. Children with hemorrhagic diathesis: correct diagnostic and therapeutic approach. *Pediatr Med Chir.* 1990 Jan-Feb;12(1):1-13.

[4] Matsunaga AT, Lubin BH. Hemolytic anemia in the newborn. *Clin Perinatol.* 1995 Sep;22(3):803-28.

[5] Zanella A, Colombo MB, Rossi F, Merati G, Sirchia G. Congenital non-spherocytic haemolytic anaemias. *Haematologica.* 1989 Jul-Aug;74(4):387-96.

[6] Weinstein L. Irregular antibodies causing hemolytic disease of the newborn: a continuing problem. *Clin Obstet Gyn*ecol. 1982 Jun;25(2):321-32.

[7] Weinstein L. Irregular antibodies causing hemolytic disease of the newborn. *Obstet Gynecol Surv.* 1976 Aug;31(8):581-91.

[8] Narang A, Jain N. Haemolytic disease of newborn. *Indian J Pediatr.* 2001 Feb;68(2):167-72.

[9] Urbaniak SJ. Alloimmunity to RhD in humans. *Transfus Clin Biol.* 2006 Mar-Apr;13(1-2):19-22.

[10] Van Kim CL, Colin Y, Cartron JP. Rh proteins: key structural and functional components of the red cell membrane. *Blood Rev.* 2006 Mar;20(2):93-110.

[11] Urbaniak SJ, Greiss MA. RhD haemolytic disease of the fetus and the newborn. *Blood Rev.* 2000 Mar;14(1):44-61.

[12] Mochizuki K, Ohto H, Hirai S, Ujiie N, Amanuma F, Kikuta A, Miura S, Yasuda H, Ishijima A, Suzuki H. Hemolytic disease of the newborn due to anti-Di: a case study and review of the literature. *Transfusion.* 2006 Mar;46(3):454-60.

[13] Mundy CA. Intravenous immunoglobulin in the management of hemolytic disease of the newborn. *Neonatal Netw.* 2005 Nov-Dec;24(6):17-24.

[14] Peterec SM. Management of neonatal Rh disease. *Clin Perinatol.* 1995 Sep;22(3):561-92.

[15] Dagoglu T, Ovali F, Samanci N, Bengisu E. High-dose intravenous immunoglobulintherapy for rhesus haemolytic disease. *J Int Med Res.* 1995 Jul-Aug;23(4):264-71.

[16] Kumpel BM.On the mechanism of tolerance to the Rh D antigen mediated by passive anti-D (Rh D prophylaxis). *Immunol Lett.* 2002 Jun 3;82(1-2):67-73.

[17] Yang SM, Wu QY, Luo HQ, Lan JC. Correlation of newborn hemolytic disease with ABO antibodies in sera of pregnant women. *Zhongguo Shi Yan Xue Ye Xue Za Zhi.* 2005 Oct;13(5):875-7.

[18] Herschel M, Karrison T, Wen M, Caldarelli L, Baron B. Isoimmunization is unlikely to be the cause of hemolysis in ABO-incompatible but direct antiglobulin test-negative neonates. *Pediatrics*. 2002 Jul;110(1 Pt 1):127-30.

[19] Waldron P, de Alarcon P. ABO hemolytic disease of the newborn: a unique constellation of findings in siblings and review of protective mechanisms in the fetal-maternal system. *Am J Perinatol.* 1999; 16(8):391-8.

[20] Han P, Kiruba R, Ong R, Joseph R, Tan KL, Wong HB. Haematolytic disease due to ABO incompatibility: incidence and value of screening in an Asian population. *Aust Paediatr J.* 1988 Feb;24(1):35-8.

[21] Levine DH, Meyer HB. Newborn screening for ABO hemolytic disease. *Clin Pediatr (Phila)*. 1985 Jul;24(7):391-4.

[22] Chen JY, Ling UP. Prediction of the development of neonatal hyperbilirubinemia in ABO incompatibility. *Zhonghua Yi Xue Za Zhi (Taipei)*. 1994 Jan;53(1):13-8.

[23] Whyte J, Graham H. Prediction of the severity of ABO haemolytic disease of the newborn by cord blood tests. *Acta Paediatr Scand.* 1981 Mar;70(2):217-22.

[24] Schonitzer D, Frisch H. Incidence, laboratory diagnosis and serologic prediction of hemolytic disease of newborn infants due to ABO incompatibility. *Padiatr Padol.* 1984; 19(3):263-78.

[25] Toy PT, Reid ME, Papenfus L, Yeap HH, Black D. Prevalence of ABO maternal-infant incompatibility in Asians, Blacks, Hispanics and Caucasians. *Vox Sang.* 1988; 54(3):181-3.

[26] Sarici SU, Yurdakok M, Serdar MA, Oran O, Erdem G, Tekinalp G, Yigit S. An early (sixth-hour) serum bilirubin measurement is useful in predicting the development of significant hyperbilirubinemia and severe ABO hemolytic disease in a selective high-risk population of newborns with ABO incompatibility. *Pediatrics.* 2002 Apr;109(4):e53.

[27] Brouwers HA, Overbeeke MA, van Ertbruggen I, Schaasberg W, Alsbach GP, van der Heiden C, van Leeuwen EF, Stoop JW, Engelfriet CP. What is the best predictor of the severity of ABO-haemolytic disease of the newborn? *Lancet.* 1988 Sep 17;2(8612):641-4.

[28] Miqdad AM, Abdelbasit OB, Shaheed MM, Seidahmed MZ, Abomelha AM, Arcala OP. Intravenous immunoglobulin G (IVIG) therapy for significant hyperbilirubinemia in ABO hemolytic disease of the newborn. *J Matern Fetal Neonatal Med.* 2004 Sep;16(3):163-6.

[29] Lakatos L, Csathy L, Nemes E. "Bloodless" treatment of a Jehovah's Witness infant with ABO hemolytic disease. *J Perinatol.* 1999 Oct-Nov;19(7):530-2.

[30] Redman CM, Lee S. The Kell blood group system. *Transfus Clin Biol.* 1995; 2(4):243-9.

[31] Lee S. Molecular basis of Kell blood group phenotypes. *Vox Sang.* 1997; 73(1):1-11.

[32] Wenk RE, Goldstein P, Felix JK. Kell alloimmunization, hemolytic disease of the newborn, and perinatal management. *Obstet Gynecol.* 1985 Oct;66(4):473-6.

[33] Bowman JM, Pollock JM, Manning FA, Harman CR, Menticoglou S. Maternal Kell blood group alloimmunization. *Obstet Gynecol.* 1992 Feb;79(2):239-44.

[34] Rodesch F, Lambermont M, Donner C, Simon P, Romasco F, Schwers J, Wybran J.Chorionic biopsy in management of severe Kell alloimmunization. *Am J Obstet Gynecol.* 1987 Jan;156(1):124-5.

[35] Caine ME, Mueller-Heubach E.Kell sensitization in pregnancy. *Am J Obstet Gynecol.* 1986 Jan;154(1):85-90.

[36] Mayne KM, Bowell PJ, Pratt GA. The significance of anti-Kell sensitization in pregnancy. *Clin Lab Haematol.* 1990;12(4):379-85.

[37] Reid ME, Sausais L, Oyen R, Storry JR, Shukla H, Hsu T, Lim SM. First example of hemolytic disease of the newborn caused by anti-Or and confirmation of the molecular basis of Or. *Vox Sang.* 2000;79(3):180-2.

[38] Pela I, Seracini D, Caprioli A, Castelletti F, Giammanco A.Hemolytic uremic syndrome in an infant following Bordetella pertussis infection. *Eur J Clin Microbiol Infect Dis.* 2006 Aug;25(8):515-7.

[39] Huang DT, Chi H, Lee HC, Chiu NC, Huang FY. T-antigen activation for prediction of pneumococcus-induced hemolytic uremic syndrome and hemolytic anemia. *Pediatr Infect Dis J.* 2006 Jul;25(7):608-10.

[40] Hsieh YC, Hsiao CH, Tsao PN, Wang JY, Hsueh PR, Chiang BL, Lee WS, Huang LM.Necrotizing pneumococcal pneumonia in children: the role of pulmonary gangrene. *Pediatr Pulmonol.* 2006 Jul;41(7):623-9.

[41] Sartori PC, Enayat MS, Darbyshire PJ. Congenital microangiopathic haemolytic anemia: a variant of thrombotic thrombocytopenic purpura?: *Pediatr Hematol Oncol.* 1993 Jul Sep;10(3):271-7.

[42] Bolde SA, Shete SS, Dantkale SS, Deshpande NM, Zawar MP. Kasabach-Merritt syndrome: a case report. *Indian J Pathol Microbiol.* 2005 Jan;48(1):27-9.

[43] Brasanac D, Janic D, Boricic I, Jovanovic N, Dokmanovic L. Retroperitoneal kaposiform hemangioendothelioma with tufted angioma-like features in an infant with Kasabach-Merritt syndrome. *Pathol Int.* 2003 Sep;53(9):627-31.

[44] Martinez AE, Robinson MJ, Alexis JB.Kaposiform hemangioendothelioma associated with nonimmune fetal hydrops. *Arch Pathol Lab Med.* 2004 Jun;128(6):678-81.

[45] Sarkar M, Mulliken JB, Kozakewich HP, Robertson RL, Burrows PE. Thrombocytopenic coagulopathy (Kasabach-Merritt phenomenon) is associated with Kaposiform hemangioendothelioma and not with common infantile hemangioma. *Plast Reconstr Surg.* 1997 Nov;100(6):1377-86.

Chapter 8

HYDROPS FETALIS AND THALSSEMIA

INTRODUCTION TO HYDROPS FETALIS

Hydrops fetalis is a totally unwanted outcome of pregnancy. Hydrops fetalis can be the results of many disorders [1-2]. It is a deadly disorder that causes fetal death. It is concluded that sonography could play a major role in determining the optimal approach to perinatal management of the fetus in hydrops fetalis, and thus contribute to a reduction in the perinatal mortality and morbidity associated with this disorder [1]. The clinical implications of fetal ascites with or without anasarca, maternal hydramnios, maternal oligohydramnios, or an abnormally thick placenta are discussed as they relate to fetal outcome [1]. The causes of hydrop fetalis may be immunological or non-immunological causes.

A. Immunological Hydrops Fetalis

Immunological hydrops fetalis is usually due to blood group incompatibility. Rh incompatibility is the major cause of immunological hydrops fetalis. In addition to general Rh incompatibility, Anti-C(w) alloimmunization can also present as hydrops fetalis [3]. In 2001, van Kamp et al performed a study to test the hypothesis that the degree of immune fetal hydrops predicts outcome in red blood cell-alloimmunized pregnancies [4]. In contrast with severe hydrops, there is a high rate of reversal of mild hydrops after adequate treatment and 98% of fetuses survived after reversal of hydrops [4]. Craparo et al a study to evaluate the effects of serial intravascular transfusions on RhD-alloimmunized fetuses with ascites/hydrops at the time of the first transfusion by measuring multiple hematological/biochemical blood variables [5]. According to this work, RhD-alloimmunized fetuses with ascites/hydrops at the time of the first transfusion had a survival rate of 87%. [5] Alterations of several biochemical fetal blood indices are present at the first sampling/transfusion, but most variables normalize with intravascular transfusions [5]. To improve the outcome of red blood cell-alloimmunized pregnancies, early diagnosis of fetal anemia and referral to a specialized center are important [4]. As a result of the advent of routine Rh screening, most cases are not currently related to Rh incompatibility [6].

Evaluation for the presence of maternal anti-D antibody should be undertaken at the first prenatal visit. First-time sensitized pregnancies are followed with serial maternal titers and, when necessary, serial amniocenteses to detect fetal bilirubin by DeltaOD(450) [7]. In cases of a heterozygous paternal genotype, new deoxyribonucleic acid techniques now make it possible to diagnose the fetal blood type through amniocentesis or even from plasma/serum deoxyribonucleic acid analysis [7]. In some situations, intrauterine transfusion is necessary through ultrasound-directed puncture of the umbilical cord with the direct intravascular injection of red cells [7]. Genetic, metabolic, chromosomal, and syndromic causes are among the most frequently identified causes of nonimmune hydrops [6]. The importance of determining the underlying cause of hydrops becomes evident once issues such as prognosis, specific treatment, and risk of recurrence are considered [6]. More details on the neonatal blood group incompatibility can be found in another chapter in this book.

B. Non-Immunological Hydrops Fetalis

There are several causes of non-immunological hydrops fetalis. These includes infections and congenital disorders. Many infections can causes hydrop fetalis due to the pathological change of many organ systems of the infected fetus especially for skeletal and cardiovascular systems. The important infection that can cause hydrops fetalis is parvovirus B19 [8]. Basically, the Parvoviridae, a family of viruses with single-stranded DNA genomes widely spread from invertebrates to mammal and human hosts, display a remarkable evolutionary capacity uncommon in DNA genomes [8-9]. Parvovirus populations show high genetic heterogeneity and large population sizes resembling the quasispecies found in RNA viruses [8-9]. These viruses multiply in proliferating cells, causing acute, persistent or latent infections relying in the immunocompetence and developmental stage of the hosts.It is confirmed that an intrauterine parvovirus B19 infection can result in severe fetal anemia and hydrops fetalis, which can lead to death [8]. The most reliable technique for diagnosis of fetal B19 infection is detection of viral DNA in fetal blood [10]. Stenner et al reported that demonstrated that following an acute parvovirus-B19-infection of the mother IgM-antibodies could be proofed for 6 - 8 (- 10) weeks [11]. On the other side parvovirus-B19-DNA in the mothers blood is detectable by means of PCR for 8 - 10 weeks and in some cases even more than 15 weeks [11]. The infection generally follows a benign course with intrauterine therapy [12]. Cordocentesis allows precise assessment of fetal anemia which can then be corrected by intravenous packed red cell transfusion [13]. Under this regimen, the outcome proved favorable in the majority of fetuses, even those that were severely anemic [13]. For untreated affected case, the neonate usually dies after intrauterine therapy and premature delivery [12]. The fetus was diagnosed with oedema, cardiomegaly, poor myocardial contractility and a pericardial effusion [12]. The post-mortem examination confirmed the hydrops and proved persistent Parvovirus infection, cardiac involvement and severe liver fibrosis [12]. Since, the condition can be diagnosed and treated antenatally and therefore should be included in the differential diagnosis of causes of hydrops fetalis [14].

Another infection that can cause hydrops fetalis is toxoplasmosis. This infection is a parasitic infection and is common in the immunocompromised host. Also, it is included as a member of TORCH agents, important transplancental infections. Many cases of hydrops fetalis due to congenital toxoplasmosis are reported [15-16]. Although uncommon, toxoplasmosis should be considered in the differential diagnosis of hydrops fetalis, particularly when the preliminary clinical work-up suggests a nonimmunologic basis for the hydrops [16]. Although the clinical outcome in an infant as severely affected as this one will remain poor, the therapy for toxoplasmosis has improved over the years, and with quick diagnosis of the disease, a less severely affected infant may have a better prognosis [16]. CMV is another TORCH agent that is reported as the corresponding agent for hydrops fetalis [17]. The autopsy findings can reveal the presence of widespread CMV disease, including pneumonitis, enteritis, and myocarditis [17].

Last but not least, the syphilis, the old infection is also another unforgettable cause of hydrops fetalis. Fetal syphilis is the presumed diagnosis when the sonographic findings of fetal hydrops are found in the presence of maternal syphilis [18-19]. Severe maceration hydrops can be seen in congenital syphilis. Despite severe maceration with visceral autolysis, spirochetes could be easily detected using Warthin-Starry stains [18]. In a patient population where prenatal care is not always obtained, and maternal serologic tests results are not available at the time of delivery, these pathologic clues are very helpful in detecting congenital syphilis in macerated stillborn fetuses where the classic findings of syphilitic infection, including hydrops fetalis and plasma cell infiltrates, may be masked [18]. Efforts to control the disease depend on the effectiveness of established screening strategies and treatment of infected pregnant women [20]. Although VDRL is routinely requested test for antenatal clinic, there are also some limitations of this test. False-negative test results can be seen and leave the fetus at risk for acquiring congenital syphilis [20]. In those cases, the false-negative results are usually caused by the prozone phenomenon [20]. Therefore, nontreponemal testing should be repeated using serum dilutions to prevent a missed diagnosis of syphilis [20]. The antenatal detection of hepatomegaly, which is probably the initial sonographic manifestation of hydrops fetalis, may ultimately identify the fetus affected with congenital syphilis [19].

The other main groups of non-immunological hydrops fetalis is congenital disorders. The most important disorders are hemoglobin disorders (thalassemia and hemoglobinopathies). The details on these diseases will be presented in the next session. In addition to the hemoglobin disorders, there are also many chromosomal disorders that can lead to hydrops fetalis. Deletion of chromosome 6 p is an example [21]. The autopsy can reveal hydrops fetalis with cleft lips, hydronephrosis of kidney or absence of kidney, spleen, and thymus gland, truncus arteriosus, and single umbilical artery [21]. Deletion of chromosome 10 is another example. The affected case is usually a hydrops with with ascites and dysmorphic facial features at birth [22].

THALASSEMIA

Thalassemia is a common congenital disorder. It can be classified as one of the most common congenital disorder in human beings. Thalassemic syndromes, characterized by anemia secondary to genetic defects of hemoglobin, are one of the most common of the genetic blood disorders in the tropics [23-25]. Basically, hemoglobin is composed of the heme and globin chains. The fundamental abnormality in thalassemia is impaired production of either the alpha or beta globin chains. The defects in thalassemia might be on alpha globin chain genes or the beta globin chain gene. Alpha thalassemia occurs when one or more of the four alpha chain genes fails to function while beta thalassemia when one or all of the two beta chain genes fails to function [23-27]. Comparing to alpha thalassemia, beta thalassemia rarely arises from the complete loss of a beta globin gene [23-27]. The beta globin gene usually presents, but produces little beta globin protein, therefore, the degree of suppression varies [23-27]. In some cases, the affected beta gene makes essentially no beta globin protein (beta-0-thalassemia) while in other cases, the production of beta chain protein is lower than normal, but not zero (beta-(+)-thalassemia) [23-27]. Similar to other inherited disorder, the defect can be detected as hemogenicity or heterogenicity. In addition, the combination between thalassemia and hemoglobinopathy is common and bring the anemia among millions of the population in the tropics. Concerning anemia in thalassemia, the microcytic type is mentioned for the non-silent carrier cases. The pathogenesis of anemia in thalassemia is complicated: many underlying causes are mentioned. The defect in red blood cell production due to the ineffective erythropoiesis can be seen and the increase of red blood cell destruction due to the hemolytic anemia and the trapping of the abnormal red blood cell by reticuloendothelial system are seen in a case with thalassemia. Concerning the ineffective erythropoiesis, marrow hyperplasia can be seen and markedly expanded marrow space lead to various skeletal manifestations including spine, skull, facial bones, and ribs [28].

A. Clinical Manifestation of Thalassemia

Clinical characteristics of the thalassemias are ineffective erythropoiesis and hemolytic anemia with microcytic-hypochromic erythrocytes [29]. However, thalassemia is very heterogeneous in the manifestation. In all thalassemias clinical features that result from anemia, transfusional, and absorptive iron overload are similar but vary in severity [28]. Briefly, the manifestation of thalassemia can be hematological system and non-hematological system manifestation. As already described, the main manifestation in hematological system is anemia. The important manifestations in non-hematological system include bone destruction, resulting in a classical sign known as thalassemic face, splenomegaly and growth retardation. Extramedullary hematopoiesis (ExmH), hemosiderosis, and cholelithiasis are among the non-skeletal manifestations of thalassemia [28]. There are also several manifestations due to the complication of thalassemia itself and treatment. Those manifestations included hemochromatosis syndrome and symptoms of several superimposed infections. However, it can be seen that most of the symptoms are usually not occur at the neonate state since the process of pathogenesis is usually chronic and the phenotypic appearance requires a long period. However, it should be noted that the previously described clinical appearances are common signs and symptoms in carriers of thalassemia. In the homozygote, which is more severe, the severe manifestation at birth as hydrops fetalis can be seen.

B. Thalassemia and Hydrops Fetalis

Hydrops fetalis can be seen in homozygous alpha thalassemia. It is called Hb Bart's hydrops fetalis. Basically, alpha-Thalassemia mutations are one of the most common mutations of man, and they cause Hb H disease and Hb Barts hydrops fetalis [30]. Fetuses with the devastating Hb Barts hydrops fetalis due to the complete lack of alpha-globin gene die in utero or shortly after birth, often during the second or third trimesters [31]. The disease burden of these syndromes and their public health importance have been largely neglected [31]. For the affected cases, alpha-Globin gene mapping of fetal DNA can confirm the diagnosis of homozygous alpha-thalassemia with deletion of all four alpha-globin genes [32]. This condition is fatal. However, there are case reports of survivor. In 2004, Joshi et al reported rhe case of a boy with hydrops fetalis who had homozygous alpha-thalassemia and alloimmune hemolytic anemia due to anti-E and anti-C blood group antibodies [33]. In this case, the patient received intrauterine red blood cell transfusions and postnatal chronic transfusion with iron chelation therapy [33]. This is the only survivor with immune- and nonimmune-induced hydrops fetalis [33].

In addition to the Hb Barts, there is also case report of hydrop fetalis due to Hb H disease.

Basically, Hb H disease is caused by deletion or inactivation of three alpha-globin genes, leaving only one intact and active alpha-globin gene. People with Hb H disease usually have moderate anemia, but are generally thought to be asymptomatic. According to the report of Chan et al, the newborn was markedly anemic, unlike those with classical Hb H disease, because the non-deletion alpha thalassemia defect is more severe than alpha thalassemia 2 [34]. Chan et al proposed that the decreased zeta genes during fetal life might have additional deleterious effects [34]. Presently, there is a described syndrome namely Hb H hydrops foetalis syndrome, caused by the inheritance of a hitherto novel alpha-globin gene point mutation (codon 35 TCC-->CCC or Serine-->Proline) and an alpha-thalassaemia deletion of the Filipino type removing all zeta-alpha-globin genes on the other chromosome 16 [35].

C. Screening for Thalassemia in Pregnancy

Basically, in endemic area, all cases with hypochromic microcytic anemia should be suspected for thalassemia disorder. The basic laboratory screenings for thalassemia are blood smear interpretation, red blood cell index determination by automated hematology analyzers, mathematical models, osmotic fragility test (OF). Of these methods, the mathematical models [36] and OF [37] are the reliable and recommended test. However, in the resource-limited settings, the blood smear interpretation is still useful [38]. In Thailand, an endemic country for thalassemic disorder, the hemoglobin electrophoresis and molecular diagnosis is proved not cost – effective [39]. For more specific test, hemoglobin electrophoresis is widely used. This test can determine the different types of hemoglobin in the blood by a electrical separating process that causes movement of particles in an electric field, resulting in formation of hemoglobin bands that separate toward one end or the other in the field. Quantitative determination of each hemoglobin band by densitometry is then performed. The hemoglobin electrophoresis is still used as a reference for diagnosis of thalassemia in the developing tropical countries. However, due to their limited resolution, incorrect or unresolved diagnosis of common hemoglobinopathies are sometimes encountered [40]. High-performance liquid chromatographic methods have been developed for either screening or confirmation of hemoglobinopathies with relatively high sensitivity or specificity [40]. The simplicity of the sample preparation, superior resolution of the method, and accurate quantitation of hemoglobin concentration, combined with complete automation, make this an ideal methodology for the routine diagnosis of hemoglobin disorders in a clinical laboratory [40]. At the present the most accurate method is mocular diagnosis. The molecular diagnosis can not only determine the type of thalassemia but also the other mutations. However, due to the fact that the cost is very high, it is not recommended for the endemic areas where are usually underdeveloped.

D. Treatment for Hb Barts Hydrops Fetalis

There are several attempts to find the proper treatment for the fetus with Hb Barts. In utero exchange transfusion is an alternative. Fung et al reported that Post-transfusion haemoglobin pattern after transfusion suggested that a total haematocrit of 0.52 may be the desired post-exchange transfusion hematocrit to aim for [41]. For the affected neonate, bone marrow transplantation (BMT) from a matched sibling is the recommended option [42]. Gene therapy is still the new hope and research focus.

HEMOGLOBINOPATHY

Hemoglobinopathy is the other group of hemoglobin disorder. Hemoglobinopathy is a group of inherited hemoglobin disorders where the structure of hemoglobin is abnormal, or where hemoglobin was improperly formed but not due to the depletion of the globin gene. Similar to thalassemia, hemoglobinopathy can lead to anemia and becomes an important anemic health problem in the tropics. Until present, there have been more than one hundred of hemoglobinopathies documented in the literature. One hemoglobinopathy has its own underlying genetic defect, therefore, has its specific property and manifestation. In this chapter, the important hemoglobinopathies that can lead to hydrops fetalis will be discussed.

A. Hemoglobin Constant Spring

Hemoglobin Constant Spring (Hb CS) is an a chain variant with an elongated alpha globin chain of 28 to 31 amino acids. This is caused by a mutation that alter the mRNA termination codon. Hb CS is common in Southeast Asia. Similar to other hemoglobinopathies, the hemoglobin electrophoreis is the definitive diagnosis for Hb CS. Concerning the hemoglobin electrophoreis, the mobility is between carbonic anhydrase and Hb A, on cellulose acetate. The percentage is usually about 1% in heterozygote carriers, 5 to

7% in homozygotes, and 3 to 5% in hemoglobin H disease caused by Hb CS with trans two gene deletion alapha thalassemia. Clinically, heterozygotes with Hb CS and two normal trans at genes are hematologically normal while homozygotes for Hb CS have a mild hemolytic anemia and may have splenomegaly [43-44]. Homozygosity of Hb CS is generally characterized with mild hemolytic anemia, jaundice, and splenomegaly. Hydrop fetalis due to Hb CS can be seen and considered as an unusual and serious in utero complication in a fetus with Hb CS/CS [45]. The affected cases usually presents with fetal anemia and hydrops. Intrauterine transfusions can be given which renders a favorable outcome [45].

B. Hemoglobin Taybe

Hemoglobin Taybe is a rare hemoglobinopathy. It an is unstable alpha-chain hemoglobin variant caused by a deletion of a threonine residue at codon 38 or 39 of the alpha-1 globin chain [46]. Most affected cases develop intrauterine hemolytic anemia, which subsequently led to hydrops fetalis [46]. Arnon et al suggested that hemoglobin Taybe should be considered in the differential diagnosis of hydrops fetalis and that known affected fetuses be carefully followed both antenatally and postnatally [46].

REFERENCES

[1] Fleischer AC, Killam AP, Boehm FH, Hutchison AA, Jones TB, Shaff MI, Barrett JM, Lindsey AM, James AE Jr. Hydrops fetalis: sonographic evaluation and clinical implications. *Radiology*. 1981 Oct;141(1):163-8.

[2] Gordon H. The diagnosis of hydrops fetalis. Clin Obstet Gynecol. 1971 Jun;14(2):548-60.

[3] Kollamparambil TG, Jani BR, Aldouri M, Soe A, Ducker DA. Anti-C(w) alloimmunization presenting as hydrops fetalis. *Acta Paediatr*. 2005 Apr;94(4):499-501.

[4] van Kamp IL, Klumper FJ, Bakkum RS, Oepkes D, Meerman RH, Scherjon SA, Kanhai HH.The severity of immune fetal hydrops is predictive of fetal outcome after intrauterine treatment. *Am J Obstet Gynecol*. 2001 Sep;185(3):668-73.

[5] Craparo FJ, Bonati F, Gementi P, Nicolini U. The effects of serial intravascular transfusions in ascitic/hydropic RhD-alloimmunized fetuses. *Ultrasound Obstet Gynecol*. 2005 Feb;25(2):144-8.

[6] Steiner RD. Hydrops fetalis: role of the geneticist. *Semin Perinatol*. 1995 Dec;19(6):516-24.

[7] Moise KJ Jr. Management of rhesus alloimmunization in pregnancy. *Obstet Gynecol*. 2002 Sep;100(3):600-11.

[8] Taksaphan S, Kleebkaew P, Komwilaisak R, Kiatchoosakun P, Jirapradittha J, Ratanasiri T. Hydrops fetalis caused by parvovirus B19 infection: case report and literature review. *J Med Assoc Thai*. 2006 Aug;89(8):1277-86.

[9] Lopez-Bueno A, Villarreal LP, Almendral JM. Parvovirus variation for disease: a difference with RNA viruses? *Curr Top Microbiol Immunol.* 2006;299:349-70.

[10] Best JM. Laboratory diagnosis of intrauterine and perinatal virus infections. *Clin Diagn Virol.* 1996 May;5(2-3):121-9.

[11] Stenner S, Enders G, Klee A, Eiden U, Weidner A, Gonser M. Urbaniak SJ, Greiss MA. RhD haemolytic disease of the fetus and the newborn. *Blood Rev.* 2000 Mar;14(1):44-61.

[12] Marton T, Martin WL, Whittle MJ. Hydrops fetalis and neonatal death from human parvovirus B19: an unusual complication. *Prenat Diagn.* 2005 Jul;25(7):543-5.

[13] Schild RL, Bald R, Plath H, Eis-Hubinger AM, Enders G, Hansmann M. Intrauterine management of fetal parvovirus B19 infection. *Ultrasound Obstet Gynecol.* 1999 Mar;13(3):161-6.

[14] Moore L, Chambers HM, Foreman AR, Khong TY. A report of human parvovirus B19 infection in hydrops fetalis. First Australian cases confirmed by serology and immunohistology. *Med J Aust.* 1993 Sep 6;159(5):344-5.

[15] Friedman S, Ford-Jones LE, Toi A, Ryan G, Blaser S, Chitayat D. Congenital toxoplasmosis: prenatal diagnosis, treatment and postnatal outcome. *Prenat Diagn.* 1999 Apr;19(4):330-3.

[16] Zornes SL, Anderson PG, Lott RL. Congenital toxoplasmosis in an infant with hydrops fetalis. *South Med J.* 1988 Mar;81(3):391-3.

[17] Sampath V, Narendran V, Donovan EF, Stanek J, Schleiss MR. Nonimmune hydrops fetalis and fulminant fatal disease due to congenital cytomegalovirus infection in a premature infant. *J Perinatol.* 2005 Sep;25(9):608-11.

[18] Young SA, Crocker DW. Occult congenital syphilis in macerated stillborn fetuses. *Arch Pathol Lab Med.* 1994 Jan;118(1):44-7.

[19] Nathan L, Twickler DM, Peters MT, Sanchez PJ, Wendel GD Jr. Fetal syphilis: correlation of sonographic findings and rabbit infectivity testing of amniotic fluid. *J Ultrasound Med.* 1993 Feb;12(2):97-101.

[20] Berkowitz K, Baxi L, Fox HE. False-negative syphilis screening: the prozone phenomenon, nonimmune hydrops, and diagnosis of syphilis during pregnancy. *Am J Obstet Gynecol.* 1990 Sep;163(3):975-7.

[21] Suwanrath-Kengpol C, Limprasert P, Mitarnun W. Prenatal diagnosis of deletion of chromosome 6p presenting with hydrops fetalis. *Prenat Diagn.* 2004 Nov;24(11):887-9.

[22] Jain R, Jones C. Hydrops fetalis in an interstitial deletion of chromosome 10. *Am J Med Genet.* 2001 Feb 1;98(4):320-3.

[23] Lo L, Singer ST. Thalassemia: current approach to an old disease. *Pediatr Clin North Am* 2002;49:1165-91.

[24] Old JM. Screening and genetic diagnosis of haemoglobin disorders. *Blood Rev* 2003;17:43-53.

[25] Fucharoen S, Wanichagoon G. Thalassemia and abnormal hemoglobin. *Int J Hematol* 2002;76 Suppl 2:83-9.

[26] Gabutti V. Current therapy for thalassemia in Italy. Ann N Y Acad Sci 1990; 612:268-74

[27] Glader BE, Look KA. Hematologic disorders in children from southeast Asia. *Pediatr Clin North Am* 1996;43:665-81.

[28] Tunaci M, Tunaci A, Engin G, Ozkorkmaz B, Dincol G, Acunas G, Acunas B. Imaging features of thalassemia. *Eur Radiol* 1999;9:1804-9.

[29] Fujita S. Congenital hemolytic anemia--hemoglobin abnormality - thalassemia. *Nippon Rinsho* 1996;54:2454-9.

[30] Chui DH. Alpha-thalassemia: Hb H disease and Hb Barts hydrops fetalis. *Ann N Y Acad Sci.* 2005;1054:25-32.

[31] Chui DH. Alpha-thalassaemia and population health in Southeast Asia. *Ann Hum Biol.* 2005 Mar-Apr;32(2):123-30.

[32] Bowman E, Watts J, Burrows R, Chui DH. Hemoglobin barts hydrops fetalis syndrome. *Haematologia (Budap).* 1987;20(3):125-30.

[33] Joshi DD, Nickerson HJ, McManus MJ. Hydrops fetalis caused by homozygous alpha-thalassemia and Rh antigen alloimmunization: report of a survivor and literature review. *Clin Med Res.* 2004 Nov;2(4):228-32.

[34] Chan V, Chan TK, Liang ST, Ghosh A, Kan YW, Todd D. Hydrops fetalis due to an unusual form of Hb H disease. *Blood.* 1985 Jul;66(1):224-8.

[35] Lorey F, Charoenkwan P, Witkowska HE, Lafferty J, Patterson M, Eng B, Waye JS, Finklestein JZ, Chui DH. Hb H hydrops foetalis syndrome: a case report and review of literature. *Br J Haematol.* 2001 Oct;115(1):72-8.

[36] Suwansaksri J, Wiwanitkit V, Paritpokee N. Screening for hemoglobin disorders in Thai pregnant women by England and Frazer's calculation method. *Arch Gynecol Obstet* 2004 Dec;270(4):211-3.

[37] Wiwanitkit V, Suwansaksri J, Paritpokee N. Combined one-tube osmotic fragility (OF) test and dichlorophenol-indolphenol (DCIP) test screening for hemoglobin disorders, an experience in 213 Thai pregnant women. *Clin Lab* 2002; 48: 525-528.

[38] Wiwanitkit V. Blood smear interpretation for screening of hemoglobin disorder in Thai pregnant women, is it effective? *Reg 4 Med J* 2000; 19: 91 – 4.

[39] Paritpokee N, SuwansaksriJ, SiritantikornA, Wiwanitkit V. Cost –effective analysis of screening tests for inherited hemoglobin disorders in pregnancies. *Chula Med J* 1999; 43: 883-891.

[40] Ou CN, Rognerud CL. Diagnosis of hemoglobinopathies: electrophoresis vs. HPLC. *Clin Chim Acta.* 2001 Nov;313(1-2):187-94.

[41] Fung TY, Lau TK, Tam WH, Li CK. In utero exchange transfusion in homozygous alpha-thalassaemia: a case report. *Prenat Diagn.* 1998 Aug;18(8):838-41.

[42] Chik KW, Shing MM, Li CK, Leung TF, Tsang KS, Yuen HL, Cheng SB, Yuen PM. Treatment of hemoglobin Bart's hydrops with bone marrow transplantation. *J Pediatr.* 1998;132(6):1039-42.

[43] Laig M, Pape M, Hundrieser J, Flatz G, Sanguansermsri T, Das BM, Deka R, Yongvanit P, Mularlee N. The distribution of the Hb constant spring gene in Southeast Asian populations. *Hum Genet* 1990 ;84:188-90.

[44] Hsia YE, Ford CA, Shapiro LJ, Hunt JA, Ching NS. Molecular screening for haemoglobin constant spring. *Lancet.* 1989;1:988-91.

[45] Charoenkwan P, Sirichotiyakul S, Chanprapaph P, Tongprasert F, Taweephol R, Sae-Tung R, Sanguansermsri T. Anemia and hydrops in a fetus with homozygous hemoglobin constant spring. *J Pediatr Hematol Oncol.* 2006 Dec;28(12):827-30.

[46] Arnon S, Tamary H, Dgany O, Litmanovitz I, Regev R, Bauer S, Dolfin T, Yacobovich J, Wolach B, Jaber L. Hydrops fetalis associated with homozygosity for hemoglobin Taybe (alpha 38/39 THR deletion) in newborn triplets. *Am J Hematol.* 2004 Jul;76(3):263-6.

Chapter 9

HEREDITARY PERSISTENCE OF FETAL HEMOGLOBIN

INTRODUCTION TO FETAL HEMOGLOBIN

Hemoglobin is an important pigment found in blood. Hemoglobin is necessary for human since it has the main function in oxygen transportation. In adults, these hemoglobin molecules make up the total hemoglobin, as follows Hb A_1: 95% to 98%, Hb A_2: 2% to 3% and Hb F: 0.8% to 2% while in children under 6 months, there are more Hb F, in new born upto 80 %. It can be seen that there is a different in amount of each hemoglobin in adult and pediatric population. In general, the bone marrow is the site for blood cell production as well as hemoglobin synthesis. However, the function of bone marrow in hemoglobin synthesis does not exist in fetal in utero [1 – 2]. The first blood cells observed in the embryo are large nucleated erythroblasts generated in blood islands of the extraembryonic yolk sac. These unique red cells have been termed primitive because of their resemblance to nucleated erythroblasts of nonmammalian species [2]. It is now widely assumed that hematopoiesis in the yolk sac is "primitive" and that "definitive" hematopoiesis has its origins in the aorta/gonad/mesonephros region [2]. Hemopoietic stem cells appear to derive from hemangioblasts that are of mesodermal origin [3]. Yolk sac milieu is permissive only for erythropoiesis which proceeds synchronously and may be erythropoietin-insensitive [3]. Yolk sac milieu is not permissive for the development of other cell lines [3]. The final product is nucleated red cells. Yolk sac hemopoiesis is an example par excellence of primitive (as compared to definitive) form of hemopoiesis [3]. Hemopoietic stem cells then seem to migrate via the bloodstream to the liver and spleen to seed these tissues, which then carry the burden of hemopoiesis until birth and for some time thereafter [3]. The important quality of fetal hemoglobin is its high oxidizability [4]. It permits the senescent fetal red cell to be hemolysed intravascularly before any membrane alterations appear [4]. The heme is dealt with by the placenta. Since no erythrophagocytosis has occurred, no bilirubin is formed. This process prevents bilirubin, which is toxic to the fetal liver, to reach it [4].

Basically, alpha-Globin synthesis is observed in the yolk sac by 3 weeks of gestation and, by 9 weeks of gestation, alpha-globin represents the main alpha-like hemoglobin in the fetus. By contrast, the switch to beta-globin chain synthesis usually remains incomplete until 1 year after birth [1]. Hemoglobin (Hb F) synthesis is high at birth, followed by a decline to adult levels by 10 months of age [5]. The individual components of the switch from embryonic to adult erythropoiesis are developmentally regulated, and their interaction with one another is complex [6]. Basic defects, such as absence of erythropoietin production, lead to early embryonic or fetal death [6]. Other defects, such as abnormalities in the switch from the fetal to adult erythropoiesis, are less catastrophic but result in hematologic abnormalities [6]. The expression of gamma-globin is controlled by a developmentally regulated transcriptional program that is recapitulated during normal erythropoiesis in the adult bone marrow [3 - 6]. In clonal cell culture, there are important findings as the followings: (a) biosynthesis of fetal hemoglobin (HbF) is markedly augmented in cultures of adult erythropoietic precursors. (b) HbF biosynthetic capabilities inversely parallel the maturational stages of adult erythropoietic precursors in the marrow, (c) the pattern of Hb synthesized by fetal erythropoietic precursors corresponds very closely to the Hb compositions in the mature erythrocytes of the donors and (d) Burst-promoting activities ather than erythropoietin appear to stimulate HbF biosynthesis by augmentation of proliferation of precursors which are programmed to produce F cells in vivo [7].

Diagnosis of Fetal Hemoglobin

Hb F can be seen in the newborn and can be identified by several methods.

Hemoglobin electrophoresis is the classical reference technique. This test can determine the different types of hemoglobin in the blood by a electrical separating process that causes movement of particles in an electric field. The pattern of Hb F in the cord blood is shown in Figure 1. Hemoglobin chromatography is another new technique. Testing by high performance liquid chromatography (HPLC) allows the actual quantification of A_2 in the presence of Hb C or Hb E. This method provides not only the identification of the aforementioned hemoglobin and variants but also an accurate quantitation of their concentrations, particularly Hb F and A2 [8].

There is another classical laboratory investigation for Hb F namely acid elusion test. Routinely, Blood samples from pregnant women and from mothers before and after delivery can be tested for the occurrence of feto-maternal bleeding using Kleihauers acid-elution technique and a counting technique described by Schneider [9]. To simplify the reading of acid eluted blood smears for fetal hemoglobin, positive and negative controls are placed side by side on a single slide [10]. Red blood cells having high Hb F content are stained a bright pink in contrast to cells devoid of Hb F which appear as ghost cells with a faint pink outline [10]. A new method for estimating Hb F levels in individual red blood cells was developed by et al [11]. According to this new modified method, cell smears are prepared using a slide maker to ensure uniform thickness and were then stained with immunofluorescence [11]. An antifading gel was applied to preserve a stable fluorescence [11]. In addition to slide method, there are methods based on other tools. For example, the HemoCue is a portable hemoglobinometer that rapidly measures hemoglobin concentration [12]. Laifer et al reported that the HemoCue accurately measured fetal hemoglobin concentration [12]. They proposed that this instrument was valuable for use with intravascular fetal transfusions [12]. Berry et al also proposed that Hemocue system is rapid and accurate for fetal hemoglobin quantitation between 18-38 weeks' gestation regardless of extremes in gestational age or hemoglobin levels [13].

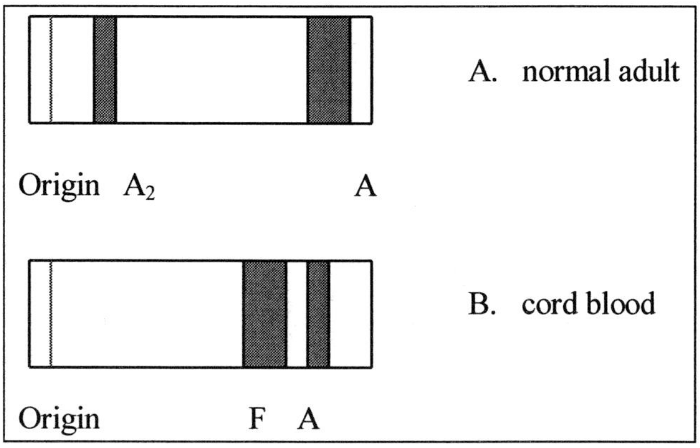

Figure 1. The electrophoresis pattern demonstrating the fetal hemoglobin (F) in B.

HEREDITARY PERSISTENCE OF FETAL HEMOGLOBIN

Hereditary persistence of fetal hemoglobin is an important hematological disorder.

The details of pathogenesis, clinical presentation, diagnosis and treatment will be further presented.

A. Pathogenesis

Hereditary persistence of fetal hemoglobin is the congenital defect in the erythropoiesis system. Beta thalassemia can be sometimes classified as a type of hereditary persistence of fetal hemoglobin. In a group of disorders called hereditary persistence of fetal hemoglobin, expression of the gamma-globin gene of HbF persists at high levels in adult erythroid cells [14]. Molecular studies of the hereditary persistence of fetal hemoglobin syndromes have identified several important regulatory elements for the normal pattern of gamma-globin gene expression [14]. Deletion as well as nondeletion types of hereditary persistence of fetal hemoglobin have been identified [14]. The nondeletion types of hereditary persistence of fetal hemoglobin are characterized by the presence of point mutations, in the promoter region of one or another gamma-globin gene, that are thought to alter interactions between various transcription factors and the promoter [14]. It is also proposed that increased activity of the hereditary persistence of fetal hemoglobin promoters may secondarily cause decreased expression of the delta- and beta-globin genes in cis possibly by competition between gamma- and beta-globin promoters for interaction with common regulatory elements [15]. The deletion types of hereditary persistence of fetal hemoglobin are thought to deregulate the normal developmental pattern of gamma-globin gene expression due to the juxtaposition of normally distant cis-acting factors into the vicinity of the gamma genes [14]. Stolle et al said that a significant mutation in HPFH-1 is the deletion of over 100 kb of genomic DNA [15]. Changsi et al proposed that high HbF production in Southeast Asian type of hereditary persistence of fetal hemoglobin occurs from a deletion of the 3'HS1 sequence and the juxtaposition of the HPFH-3 enhancer downstream to the delta-globin gene [16]. In Southeast Asia, The compound heterozygosity of beta-thalassemia and hereditary persistence of Hb F causes the phenotype of thalassemia intermedia; in contrast, homozygotes for this anomaly show only mild microcytic anemia [17].

B. Clinical presentation

Hereditary persistence of fetal hemoglobin is an autosomal co-dominant, rare, inherited condition. It occurs due to failure of switching off of the production of gamma-chains during the neonatal period leading to a high level of fetal hemoglobin in adult life but without any anemia [18].

C. Diagnosis

The diagnosis of hereditary persistence of fetal hemoglobin can be performed by identification of HbF as previously mentioned. It should be noted that high frequencies of deltabeta-thalassemia and hereditary persistence of fetal hemoglobin can be seen in endemic areas such as Thailand, therefore, there is the need for differential diagnostic methods since the hematologic parameters associated with the conditions are very similar and overlap [19]. The molecular diagnosis is the definite diagnosis tool for this condition. There is an interesting observation in the co-presentation of hereditary persistence of fetal hemoglobin with beta thalassemia. Garner et al found that beta-thalassaemia subjects with heterocellular hereditary persistence of fetal hemoglobin had higher MCV and MCH values, concomitant with lower levels of Hb A2, and a reduced ineffective erythropoiesis [20]. They conclude that co-inheritance of heterocellular hereditary persistence of fetal hemoglobin leads to a primary increase in gamma-chain synthesis in beta-thalassaemia trait and can be another confounding factor in the use of red cell indices and Hb A2 levels in population screening for beta-thalassaemia [20].

D. Treatment

Hereditary persistence of fetal hemoglobin has typically been ascribed to mutations in the beta-globin gene cluster. Pharmacologic agents, including the short-chain fatty acid butyrate, have been shown to upregulate fetal and embryonic globin gene expression [21]. Miller et al demonstrated that interferon (IFN) -gamma was an environmental factor that influences gamma-globin gene expression in the beta hemoglobinopathies in vitro [22]. They found that HbF content (expressed as picograms HbF/cell) was decreased in samples co-cultured with

IFN, increased in cultures with L-alpha-amino-n-butyric acid, but remained at control values in cultures treated with IFN plus L-alpha-amino-n-butyric acid [22]. Gene therapy is the new hope in the treatment of hereditary persistence of fetal hemoglobin. It is noted that that the 3'-juxtaposed region position exerted a positional effect associated with activation of fetal gene in hereditary persistence of fetal hemoglobin [23]. In a recent study by Wiwanitkit [24], computer prediction and gene homology programs was used to reveal gene homologues to this area. The identified gene can be a considerable point in gene therapy [24]. The results of in silico analysis of the breakpoint revealed 3 most highly homologuegenes (alignment score between 50 and 80) including a) Homo sapiens G-g globin and A-g globin genes, b) Homo sapiens b globin region (HBB@) on chromosome 11 and c) Homo sapiens chromosome 11, clone CTD-2643I7 [24].

Delta Beta Thalassemia

Physiologically, each alpha globin gene produces only about half the quantity of protein of a single beta globin gene, bringing the equality in the production of protein subunits [25 – 31]. Thalassemia occurs when a globin gene fails, and the production of globin protein subunits is imbalance [25 – 31]. As already described, the abnormality in alpha globin gene results in the whole gene detect while abnormality in beta globin chain gene can be either the whole or partial gene defect [25 – 31]. Comparing to alpha thalassemia, beta thalassemia rarely arises from the complete loss of a beta globin gene [25 - 29]. The beta globin gene usually presents, but produces little beta globin protein, therefore, the degree of suppression varies [25 - 29]. In some cases, the affected beta gene makes essentially no beta globin protein (beta-0-thalassemia) while in other cases, the production of beta chain protein is lower than normal, but not zero (beta-(+)-thalassemia) [25 - 27].

A. Basic Information on Genotype and Phenotype Correlation of Beta Thalassemia

The classical phenotype of heterozygous beta-thalassemia may be modified by a number of environmental and genetic interacting factors--among which the most relevant are: (1) coinheritance of alpha-thalassemia, which may normalize the red blood cell indices; (2) the presence of a mild beta-thalassemia mutation; (3) cotransmission of delta-thalassemia which may reduce the increase of HbA2 typical of heterozygous beta-thalassemia to normal values and (4) the presence of a silent mutation which can be defined only by imbalanced beta-globin chain synthesis [32]. Basically, two gene beta thalassemia type produces a severe anemia and a potentially life-threatening condition. The severity of the disorder depends in part on the combination of genes that have been inherited (beta 0/ beta 0; beta 0/ beta +; beta +/ beta +), therefore, some cases can be survival and becomes the problematic cases. In cases with beta 0/ beta 0, there will be no beta globin and there will be only HbF. In beta thalassemia, co-inheritance of alpha thalassemia genes such as alpha thalasemia 2 or alpha thalassemia 1 reduce the imbalance alpha/beta synthesis leading to less clinical severity [32 -

33].Fucharoen and Winichagoon noted that co-inheritance of alpha-thalassemia alleviated the severity of beta-thalassemia disease in patients with at least one allele of mild beta-thalassemia genotype [33]. This principle is known as numeric allelic principle. Bases on the allelic numeric principle, it is believed that co-inheritance of beta thalassemia with normal alpha (__/__, 4 alpha genes) can lead to more severe disease than that co-inheritance with alpha thalassemia trait (__/_-, 3 alpha genes; and _-/_- or __/--, 2 alpha genes). However, for the combination between triplicated alpha genes with beta thalassemia trait, the allelic numeric principle cannot be applied. Here, the author suggests that the control is for the entire locus-that is for the combination of alphas in a proportionate fashion to the beta chains. The issue really evolves around the cross over alpha thalassemia were three alpha genes are on one chromosome and one on the other chromosome in association with beta-thalassemia. Indeed, due to a recent genotype study by Ma et al, five copies of alpha-globin genes (alphaalphaalpha/alphaalpha) could be detected and this implies that production might be straight forward in a single alpha gene on one chromosome [34]. However, allelic proportional model is limited to explain for the other types of combination. For example, the calculations do not take in to account the experimental evidence suggesting that the deletion of one (alpha) gene results in an upregulation of the remaining genes in the same cluster.

B. What is Delta Beta Thalassemia?

Delta beta thalassemia is a variant of beta thalassemia. Since the gene encoding delta globin chain production is located very close to the beta globin gene on chromosome 11, if one gene is deleted then the other may be affected. Homozygous delta beta thalassemia is very severe and can present only Hb F similar to two gene beta thalassemia. Heterozygous delta beta thalassemia is similar to beta thalassemia but symptoms are milder. However, most patients survive to adult life with minimal transfusion requirements. The pattern of hemoglobin electrophoresis usually shows decreased Hb A and increased Hb F upto 15 %. According to the study of Cao et al, the delta beta carriers, although in many respects showing the usual picture of delta beta-thalassaemia, such as abnormal red cell indices, normal Hb A2, Hb F heterogeneously distributed in the erythrocytes, and low beta/alpha synthetic ratios, had unusually high levels of Hb F (range 10 to 20%) and particularly low glycine content (range 0.02 to 0.14 residues) in the isolated gamma CB3 peptide [35]. It should be noted that interaction of beta thalassaemia with delta beta thalassaemia occurred in children producing a clinical condition which is somewhat less severe than that of homozygous beta thalassaemia [36]. There are two main groups of delta beta thalassemia, G gamma-delta beta thalassemia and G gamma A gamma-delta beta thalassemia [37 - 38]. Hb F, which is the only Hb component in the homozygotes, has equal quantities of Ggamma and Agamma chains as in B gamma A gamma-delta beta thalassemia.The clinical and some of the hematological findings aree milder in the G gamma-delta 0 beta 0-thalassemia homozygote than in the G gamma A gamma-delta 0 beta 0-thalassemia homozygote [37].

C. Delta Beta Thalassemia and Hereditary Persistence of Fetal Hemoglobin

Ottolenghi et al suggested that the deletion of a region centered at a cluster of repetitive sequences approximately 3.5 kilobases 5' to the delta-globin gene might be critical for the persistent expression of high levels of gamma-globin in hereditary persistence of fetal hemoglobin compared to delta beta-thalassemia [39]. The concept that the deletion or mutation of specific areas (rather than nonspecific changes brought about by large deletions in the globin cluster) is important in determining the persistent expression of gamma-globin genes is supported by the finding of a nondeletion type of delta beta-thalassemia [39]. Losekoot et al found that heterozygosity for the heterocellular hereditary persistence of fetal hemoglobin brougt about a moderate (3.4% to 8.24%) increase of hemoglobin (Hb) F having a G gamma/A gamma ratio of 4:1, whereas carriers of the G gamma + ((A) gamma delta beta)(0)-thal deletion showed in their peripheral blood a considerably higher (15%) percentage of Hb F [40]. Comparison of the cases with G gamma Agamma-delta beta-thalassemia homozygotes and with G gamma A gamma- hereditary persistence of fetal hemoglobin homozygotes indicates the possibility that the proliferation of F-cell precursors may be defective in delta beta-thalassemia [41]. Both G gamma Agamma-delta beta-thalassemia homozygotes and G gamma A gamma- hereditary persistence of fetal hemoglobin homozygotes defects interact in the compound heterozygotes for G gamma A gamma delta beta 0- thalassemia and delta 0- hereditary persistence of fetal hemoglobin producing a further increase (up to 24%) of fetal hemoglobin consisting entirely of G gamma chains [40]. In addition, the possible contribution of heterocellular hereditary persistence of fetal hemoglobin to the less severe expression of the compound delta beta/beta(+)-thalassaemia heterozygosity is also reported [41]. The affected cases may healthy and never need blood transfusions [41]. The importance of the coexistence of hereditary persistence of fetal hemoglobin determinants capable of increasing the size of the F-cell population in patients affected by homozygous thalassemia is mentioned, considering the sensible benefit which derives from enhanced Hb F production in this syndrome [42].

References

[1] Olivieri NF. Fetal erythropoiesis and the diagnosis and treatment of hemoglobin disorders in the fetus and child. *Semin Perinatol.* 1997 Feb;21(1):63-9.

[2] McGrath KE, Palis J. Hematopoiesis in the yolk sac: more than meets the eye. *Exp Hematol.* 2005 Sep;33(9):1021-8.

[3] Tavassoli M. Embryonic and fetal hemopoiesis: an overview. *Blood Cells.* 1991;17(2):269-81

[4] Bogair N. The Bessis reticular cell, the hemoglobin 'switch' and the role of fetal hemoglobin: a hypothesis. *Med Hypotheses.* 1991 Feb;34(2):105-10.

[5] Pace BS, Zein S. Understanding mechanisms of gamma-globin gene regulation to develop strategies for pharmacological fetal hemoglobin induction. *Dev Dyn.* 2006 Jul;235(7):1727-37.

[6] Dame C, Juul SE. The switch from fetal to adult erythropoiesis. *Clin Perinatol.* 2000 Sep;27(3):507-26.

[7] Ogawa M, Porter PN. Fetal hemoglobin biosynthesis in clonal cell culture. *Tex Rep Biol Med.* 1980-1981;40:55-65.

[8] Ou CN, Rognerud CL. Diagnosis of hemoglobinopathies: electrophoresis vs. HPLC. 1: *Clin Chim Acta* 2001;313:187-94.

[9] Jorgensen J. Feto-maternal bleeding. During pregnancy and at delivery. *Acta Obstet Gynecol Scand.* 1977;56(5):487-90.

[10] Barr JK, Shafer JA. Preparation and storage of control slides for fetal hemoglobin determination by acid elution. *Am J Med Technol.* 1976 Jan;42(1):54-6.

[11] Horiuchi K, Osterhout ML, Kamma H, Bekoe NA, Hirokawa KJ. Estimation of fetal hemoglobin levels in individual red cells via fluorescence image cytometry. *Cytometry.* 1995 Jul 1;20(3):261-7.

[12] Laifer SA, Kuller JA, Hill LM. Rapid assessment of fetal hemoglobin concentration with the HemoCue system. *Obstet Gynecol.* 1990 Oct;76(4):723-4.

[13] Berry SM, Dombrowski MP, Blessed WB, Bichalski JA, Jones TB, Cotton DB. Fetal hemoglobin quantitations using the Hemocue system are rapid and accurate. *Obstet Gynecol.* 1993 Mar;81(3):417-20.

[14] Forget BG. Molecular basis of hereditary persistence of fetal hemoglobin. *Ann N Y Acad Sci.* 1998 Jun 30;850:38-44.

[15] Ottolenghi S, Mantovani R, Nicolis S, Ronchi A, Giglioni B. DNA sequences regulating human globin gene transcription in nondeletional hereditary persistence of fetal hemoglobin. *Hemoglobin.* 1989;13(6):523-41.

[16] Stolle CA, Penny LA, Ivory S, Forget BG, Benz EJ Jr. Sequence analysis of the gamma-globin gene locus from a patient with the deletion form of hereditary persistence of fetal hemoglobin. *Blood.* 1990 Jan 15;75(2):499-504.

[17] Changsri K, Akkarapathumwong V, Jamsai D, Winichagoon P, Fucharoen S. Molecular mechanism of high hemoglobin F production in Southeast Asian-type hereditary persistence of fetal hemoglobin. *Int J Hematol.* 2006 Apr;83(3):229-37.

[18] Trachoo O, Sura T, Sakuntabhai A, Singhasivanon P, Krudsood S, Phimpraphi W, Krasaesub S, Chanjarunee S, Looareesuwan S. Molecular characterization of hereditary persistence of fetal hemoglobin in the Karen people of Thailand. *Hemoglobin.* 2003 May;27(2):97-104.

[19] Balgir RS. Hereditary persistence of foetal haemoglobin in a tribal family of Orissa, India. *Natl Med J India.* 2004 May-Jun;17(3):138-40.

[20] Panyasai S, Fucharoen S, Surapot S, Fucharoen G, Sanchaisuriya K. Molecular basis and hematologic characterization of deltabeta-thalassemia and hereditary persistence of fetal hemoglobin in Thailand. *Haematologica.* 2004 Jul;89(7):777-81.

[21] Garner C, Dew TK, Sherwood R, Rees D, Thein SL. Heterocellular hereditary persistence of fetal haemoglobin affects the haematological parameters of beta-thalassaemia trait. *Br J Haematol.* 2003 Oct;123(2):353-8.

[22] Little JA, Dempsey NJ, Tuchman M, Ginder GD.Metabolic persistence of fetal hemoglobin. *Blood.* 1995 Apr 1;85(7):1712-8.

[23] Miller BA, Olivieri N, Hope SM, Faller DV, Perrine SP. Interferon-gamma modulates fetal hemoglobin synthesis in sickle cell anemia and thalassemia. *J Interferon Res.* 1990 Aug;10(4):357-66.

[24] Poncz M, Sutton M, Delgrosso K, Schwartz E, Surrey S. DNA methylation in hereditary persistence of fetal hemoglobin (HPFH-2). *Nucleic Acids Res* 1987; 15: 5169-79.

[25] Wiwanitkit V. Identification of putative genes for hereditary persistence of fetal hemoglobin (HPFH) *Gene Ther Mol Biol Vol* 2005; 9: 325-326.

[26] Lo L, Singer ST. Thalassemia: current approach to an old disease. *Pediatr Clin North Am* 2002;49:1165-91.

[27] Old JM. Screening and genetic diagnosis of haemoglobin disorders. *Blood Rev* 2003;17:43-53.

[28] Fucharoen S, Wanichagoon G. Thalassemia and abnormal hemoglobin. *Int J Hematol* 2002;76 Suppl 2:83-9.

[29] Gabutti V. Current therapy for thalassemia in Italy. *Ann N Y Acad Sci* 1990; 612:268-74.

[30] Glader BE, Look KA. Hematologic disorders in children from southeast Asia. *Pediatr Clin North Am* 1996;43:665-81.

[31] Giardina P, Hilgartner M. Update on thalassemia. *Pediatr Rev* 1992;13:55-62.

[32] Rund D, Rachmilewitz E. Thalassemia major 1995: older patients, new therapies. *Blood Rev* 1995; 9:25-32.

[33] Cao A, Galanello R, Rosatelli MC. Genotype-phenotype correlations in beta thalassemias. *Blood Rev.* 1994 Mar;8(1):1-12.

[34] Fucharoen S, Winichagoon P. Clinical and hematologic aspects of hemoglobin beta-thalassemia. *Curr Opin Hematol* 2000;7:106-12.

[35] Ma SK, Au WY, Chan AY, Chan LC. Clinical phenotype of triplicated alpha-globin genes and heterozygosity for beta0-thalassemia in Chinese subjects. *Int J Mol Med.* 2001;8:171-5.

[36] Cao A, Melis MA, Galanello R, Angius A, Furbetta M, Giordano P, Bernini LF. Delta beta (F)-thalassaemia in Sardinia. *J Med Genet.* 1982 Jun;19(3):184-92.

[37] Efremov GD, Nikolov N, Duma H, Schroeder WA, Miller A, Huisman TH. Delta Beta-Thalassaemia in two yugoslavian families. *Scand J Haematol.* 1975 May;14(3):226-32.

[38] Dincol G, Altay C, Aksoy M, Gurgey A, Felice AE, Huisman TH. Clinical and hematological evaluation of two delta 0 beta 0-thalassemia homozygotes. *Hemoglobin.* 1981;5(2):153-64.

[39] Amin AB, Pandya NL, Diwin PP, Darbre PD, Kattamis C, Metaxatou-Mavromati A, White JM, Wood WG, Clegg JB, Weatherall DJ. A comparison of the homozygous states for G gamma and G gamma A gamma delta beta thalassaemia. *Br J Haematol.* 1979 Dec;43(4):537-48.

[40] Ottolenghi S, Giglioni B, Taramelli R, Comi P, Mazza U, Saglio G, Camaschella C, Izzo P, Cao A, Galanello R, Gimferrer E, Baiget M, Gianni AM. Molecular comparison of delta beta-thalassemia and hereditary persistence of fetal hemoglobin DNAs: evidence of a regulatory area? *Proc Natl Acad Sci U S A.* 1982 Apr;79(7):2347-51.

[41] Reyes GR, Pina-Camara A, Felice AE, Gravely ME, Huisman TH. Delta beta-thalassemia in a Mexican family: clinical differences among homozygotes. *Hemoglobin.* 1978;2(6):513-29.

[42] Cianetti L, Care A, Sposi NM, Giampaolo A, Calandrini M, Petrini M, Massa A, Marinucci M, Mavilio F, Ceccanti M, et al. Association of heterocellular HPFH, beta(+)-thalassaemia, and delta beta(0)-thalassaemia: haematological and molecular aspects. *J Med Genet.* 1984 Aug;21(4):263-7.

[43] Marinucci M, Mavilio F, Giuliani A, Gabbianelli M, Tentori L Jr, Tentori L, Zorini CO, Lamberti E, Palazzolo A, Lanzo D. beta Thalassemia associated with increased HB F production. Evidence for the existence of a heterocellular hereditary persistence of fetal hemoglobin (HPFH) determinant linked to beta thalassemia in a southern Italian population. *Hemoglobin.* 1981;5(1):1-17.

Chapter 10

BLOOD CELL ENZYMATIC DEFICIENCY

RED BLOOD CELL ENZYMATIC DEFICIENCY

Red blood cell enzymatic deficiency is an important group of hematological disorders. The important disorders are glucose-6-phosphate dehydrogenase deficiency and pyruvate kinase deficiency. In this chapter, the details of these important red blood cell enzymatic deficiencies will be presented.

A. Glucose-6-Phosphate Dehydrogenase Deficiency

Glucose-6-phosphate dehydrogenase (G-6-PD) deficiency is an important congenital disorder. Glucose-6-phosphate dehydrogenase (G6PD, EC1.1.1.49) is an enzyme expressed in all tissues, where it catalyses the first step in the pentose phosphate pathway [1-3]. This first reaction in the pathway leads to the production of pentose phosphates and reducing power in the form of NADPH for reductive biosynthesis and maintenance of the cellular redox state [1- 3]. The defect of this enzyme namely G6PD deficiency is the most common sex linked inherited enzymatic defect, affecting over 400 million persons worldwide [1-3]. This disorder can cause hemolytic anemia [1]. The severe hemolysis and hemostatic change sometimes due to an identifiable chemical trigger, drugs or to infection [1-2]. Several widely used drugs in the tropics, especially antimalarial drugs, can induce hemolysis in the patients with G6PD deficiency. G6PD deficiency is prevalent throughout tropical and subtropical regions of the world because of the protection it affords during malaria infection [3]. G6PD plays a key role in the generation of NADPH which is essential for maintaining glutathione in the reduce state, and in the production of ribose 5-phosphate for the synthesis of nucleotides [1-4]. G6PD in its active form is either a dimer or tetramer consisting identical subunits [1-4]. It is already known that the cause of G6PD deficiency is due to the enzymatic defect at the gene level. The glucose-6-phosphate dehydrogenase (G6PD) gene is X-linked. The gene for G6PD is located on the X chromosome [4]. Human red cell G6PD consists of 515 amino acids with a molecular weight of 59,265 daltons [4]. There are numerous mutations that cause a deficiency of this enzyme in erythrocytes [5]. DNA sequence analysis has shown that the vast majority of these are caused by single amino acid substitutions [1-3]. Beutler said that different mutations, each characteristic of certain populations, were found, and had been characterized at the deoxyribonucleic acid (DNA) level [5].

The G6PD deficiency is an inheritable, X-linked recessive disorder whose primary effect is the reduction of the enzyme G6PD in red blood cells, causing destruction of the cells, called hemolysis [6]. Due to the nature of inheritance, the disease is more common in male. The hemolytic anemia in G6PD deficiency can be divided into either acute hemolytic or a chronic spherocytic type. The most well known condition is flavism. Favism is an acute hemolytic syndrome occurring in G6PD deficient individuals, about 20 %, after the consumption of fava beans [7]. The erythrocytes in affected individuals have insufficient reducing power against toxic peroxydes and free radicals generated during metabolism [8]. Normally, affected individuals are without signs of disease, but under the influence of oxidants severe intravascular hemolysis may occur [8]. One of the most important oxidants is the fava bean which, when ingested, may cause acute favism, a condition which has a 10% mortality if not treated properly [8]. Mareni *et al* noted that since not all G6PD deficient subjects were sensitive to fava beans, the possibility haf been suggested that extra erythrocytic factors might play an important role in the susceptibility to haemolytic favism [9]. They performed a study to test the hypothesis that an autosomal enzyme was involved in the pathogenesis of favism by carring out a beta-glucosidase assay in small intestine biopsies from normal subjects and G6PD deficient subjects with or without favism [9]. They found that beta-glucosidase might be involved in the absorption and metabolism of fava beans and a quantitative polymorphism could explain the different susceptibility to fava beans of G6PD deficient subjects, however, their observation showed no consistent quantitative polymorphism of beta-glucosidase in the subjects examined [9]. Damonte *et al* reported that exposure of G6PD-deficient erythrocytes in vitro to autoxidizing divicine, a pyrimidine aglycone strongly implicated in the pathogenesis of favism which leads to late accumulation of intracellular calcium, caused: (i) a marked inactivation of calcium ATPase, without changes in the molecular mass of 134 kD; and (ii) the concomitant loss of spectrin, band 3 and band 4.1, all known substrates of the calcium activated procalpain-calpain proteolytic system, thus, the increased intraerythrocytic calcium apparently results in the degradation of calcium ATPase observed in some favic patients [10]. Damonte *et al* proposed that both enhanced calcium permeability and a calcium-stimulated degradation of the calcium pump were the mechanisms responsible for the perturbation of erythrocyte calcium homeostasis in favism [10]. However, flavism is not common in the tropics. Recently, Kitayaporn *et al* proposed that G6PD deficiency and fava bean consumption do not produce hemolysis in Thailand [11]. They concluded that this might be due to the presence of different G6PD mutants to those found elsewhere or due to different consumption patterns of fava beans among the Thais compared to people in other areas with high prevalence of G6PD deficiency [11].

Although the clinical manifestation in the general population of G6PD deficiency usually relates to the exposure to triggers such as drugs, the start of manifestation in the neonate is different. In neonate, the G6PD usually manifests as neonatal jaundice due to the stress without specific triggers. G6PD is an important risk factor in the pathogenesis of severe neonatal hyperbilirubinemia [12]. Many of the recently reported cases of kernicterus, even in countries with a low overall incidence of the G-6-PD deficiency such as the United States and Canada, have been found to be enzyme deficient [12]. The G6PD subtype is also important determinant for jaundice occurrence. According to a recent published work by Wiwanitkit [13], G6PD Viangchan exhibited a stronger contribution, some 2 times, to neonatal jaundice than G6PD Canton. However, there are some reports on G6PD attack in neonate due to the exposure to external triggers. In 1995, Corchia et al reported a case of favism in a female newborn infant with G6PD deficiency whose mother had ingested fava beans 5 days before delivery [14].

Screening for G6PD deficiency is somewhat useful in the area with highly endemicity. Chuu *et al* recently indicated that severe neonatal jaundice can be effectively prevented by neonatal screening for G-6-PD deficiency [15]. Wiwanitkit also recommended the G6PD screening in combination with ABO blood group and Rh blood group as a basic screening test for the neonates with unexplained pathological hyperbilirubinemia [16]. Pao et al proposed that neonatal screening for G6PD deficiency was a useful test for preventing and early treatment of complications associated with it [17]. Chuu et al proposed that the primary consideration to include G6PD deficiency in neonatal screening program was the public health burden of G6PD deficiency associated neonatal jaundice in the target population, however, the prevalence of G6PD deficiency per se could not be the sole index of the public health burden of G6PD deficiency associated neonatal jaundice [18]. Chuu et al noted that the effectiveness of neonatal screening programs for G6PD deficiency to prevent severe neonatal jaundice had been shown based on historical comparison [18]. The classical qualitative hematology test for G-6-PD deficiency screening is methaemoglobin reduction test (MRT): an examination on color change of deficient red cell [18]. The basis of this in-vitro test is a coloric reaction using sodium nitrite and methylene blue chloride reagent [18]. Color change of blood was assessed qualitatively [18]. Diagnosis of G6PD deficiency was made if the sample was to dark brown [19]. The sensitivity of this test from the previous study is 85.7 % [19]. Recently, Sanpawat *et al* performed a comparative study between the MRT and the G6PD activity assay, a quantitative test using enzymatic principle, and reported a higher sensitivity for G6PD activity assay [19]. High specificity (98 - 100 %) of both tests was presented [19]. Recently, Wiwanikit reported that the G-6-PD activity assay was less cost effective than the methaemoglobin reduction test in screening for G6PD deficiency [20].

Basically, in the attacked G6PD cases with post-stimulated hemolysis, the treatment is necessary. The general principles of anemia management, increase red blood cell production, decrease red blood cell destruction and red blood cell replacement are recommended. In the extremely severe cases as those with flavism, the prompt treatment is necessary. The unwanted complication, tissue hypoperfusion, which can lead to cellular oxidative and peroxidative damage due to biochemical disorders in the oxygen and substrate metabolism, should be controlled [21]. Transfusion therapy is recommended in cases with severely illness. However, treatment by blood transfusion is usually supportive while effective therapy directed to treat the underlying cause of hemolysis, getting rid of the trigger, is needed [22]. However, since in neonates with attack, there is no overt trigger, therefore, the management can be only control of hemolytic anemia and prevent for the important complication hyperbilirubinemia. In very severe case, exchange transfusion should be considered. The management of hyperbilirubinemia can be found in another chapter in this book. For the correction of anemia, erythrocyte transfusion may be needed.

B. Pyruvate Kinase Deficiency

Pyruvate kinase deficiency is another important red blood cell enzymatic deficiency. Red cell pyruvate kinase deficiency is the most frequent enzyme abnormality of the glycolytic pathway [23-25]. Pyruvate kinase is a key glycolytic enzyme and has two structural genes; the L/R-gene encodes the L- and R-type PK, whereas the M-gene encodes the M1- and M2-type isozymes [26]. The isozyme switches from the M2 to the R-type during erythroid differentiation, and recent results showed that the switching was achieved by activation of the R-PK promoter activity and the involvement of erythroid-specific transcription factors has been demonstrated [26]. Glycolysis is a major energy source for red cells, therefore, PK deficiency results in hemolysis [26]. Pyruvate kinase deficiency is a congenital disorder similar to G6PD deficiency. Pyruvate kinase deficiency is the second-most common hereditary nonspherocytic hemolytic anemia [23]. The degree of haemolysis varies widely, ranging from very mild or fully compensated forms, to life-threatening neonatal anaemia and jaundice necessitating exchange transfusions. Erythrocyte pyruvate kinase is synthesized under the control of the PK-LR gene located on chromosome 1 [24]. To date, more than 150 different mutations in the PK-LR gene have been associated with pyruvate kinase deficiency [24]. Of several mutations, 1529A and 1456T being considered to be the most common mutations in Caucasians [27].

Clinical symptoms of pyruvate kinase deficiency usually occurring in compound heterozygotes for two mutant alleles and in homozygotes. The severity of haemolysis is highly variable, ranging from very mild or fully compensated forms to life-threatening neonatal anaemia necessitating exchange transfusions. Neonatal hyperbilirubinemia due to pyruvate kinase deficiency is important in neonatology [28]. The initial approach involved rapid evaluation, phototherapy, and close monitoring of serum bilirubin levels [28]. Follow-up included maintenance on folic acid, monitoring blood counts, and educating the parents about the course of pyruvate kinase deficiency, especially aplastic crisis [28].In severe rare cases of pyruvate kinase deficiency, hydrops fetalis can be the results [29]. Zanella et al reported that clinical manifestations of red cell enzyme defects are not merely dependent on the molecular properties of the mutant protein but rather reflect the complex interactions of additional factors, including genetic background, concomitant functional polymorphisms of other enzymes, posttranslational or epigenetic modifications, ineffective erythropoiesis and differences in splenic function [30].

Prompt fetal diagnosis of pyruvate kinase deficiency is feasible and allows better management of this disorder [31]. The widely used techniques are based on molecular diagnostic methods. Prenatal testing for pyruvate kinase deficiency is often requested by parents who already have an affected child. Two different approaches were used. The first, using a direct method of PCR amplification and restriction endonuclease analysis, detected mutations in fetus genomic DNA [32]. The second method, using two polymorphic sites linked to the PKRL gene, enabled us to establish which chromosome had been inherited from each parent [32].

C. Hexokinase Deficiency

Hexokinase deficiency is a rare red blood cell enzyme deficiency. This deficiency is associated with hereditary non-spherocytic haemolytic anemia [33]. To date, only 17 affected families have been reported. Human HK has four major isozymes, each of which is encoded by a separate gene [33]. Recent studies have shown that both ubiquitously expressed type I HK (HK-I) and erythroid-specific HK-R are expressed in erythrocytes, and that these isozymes are encoded by the single HK-I gene [33]. The human HK-I gene has 19 exons, the HK-I and HK-R transcripts being produced by using two distinct promoters [33]. HK-R unfolds major HK activity in immature RBCs and is rapidly degraded during the maturation process. HK-I has a porin-binding domain in its N-terminus [34]. Recent studies have shown that HK isozymes with a porin-binding domain play a role in mitochondrial integrity, suggesting that HK-I-deficient erythroid cells might be eliminated by apoptosis [34]. It is most likely that red blood cells are most labile as a result of HK-I/R deficiency since the HK-I gene but not the other isozyme genes are expressed in fetal and adult red blood cells [34]. Nonspherocytic hemolytic anemia is an important manifestation of hexokinase deficiency in neonate [35-36].

White Blood Cell Enzymatic Deficiency

Similar to red blood cell deficiency, congenital white blood cell enzymatic deficiency can also be seen. For both polymorphonuclear and monnuclear types of white blood cell, enzymatic deficiency can be seen. Important deficiencies will be further discussed.

A. Neutrophil Enzymatic Deficiency

The two common neutrophil enzymatic deficiencies are pyruvate kinase deficiency and myeloperoxidase deficiency. Neutrophil pyruvate kinase deficiency manifests different from red blood cell pyruvate kinase deficiency. Neutrophil pyruvate kinase deficiency usually presented with frequent infections [37-38]. The importance of this deficiency in the neonatal period is not much. Considering myeloperoxidase deficiency, the impairment of phagocytosis activity of neutrophil can be the result and frequent infection is the common manifestation [39]. Basically, myeloperoxidase, an iron-containing heme protein localized in the azurophilic granules of neutrophil granulocytes and in the lysosomes of monocytes, is involved in the killing of several micro-organisms and foreign cells, including bacteria, fungi, viruses, red cells, and malignant and nonmalignant nucleated cells [39-40]. Despite the primary role of the oxygen-dependent myeloperoxidase system in the destruction of certain phagocytosed microbes, subjects with total or partial myeloperoxidase deficiency generally do not have an increased frequency of infections, probably because other myeloperoxidase - independent mechanisms for microbicidal activity compensate for the lack of myeloperoxidase [39-40]. Recent interest in myeloperoxidase has extended well beyond the domain of innate host defense against infection and includes generalized inflammatory diseases, atherosclerosis, and degenerative neurologic diseases [41]. Search of the various data banks using the cDNA sequence for myeloperoxidase has uncovered previously unsuspected relationships among peroxidatively active proteins in widely different species [41]. In addition, application of the analytical tools of cell and molecular biology has allowed definition of specific genotypes underlying myeloperoxidase deficiency and the impact of particular mutations on the fate of myeloperoxidase precursors along the biosynthetic pathway [41]. Infants, children, and young adults who suffer chronic and recurrent bacterial or fungal infection despite adequate numbers of circulating granulocytes and normal or elevated levels of immunoglobulins should be suspected of having fundamental defects in granulocyte functioning especially for myeloperoxidase deficiency [42-43].

B. Eosinophil Enzymatic Deficiency

Similar to neutrophil, eosinophil myeloperoxidase deficiency can be seen. The enzyme deficit can be classified as total (negative cytochemical reactions and absence of dimethylaminoazobenzene-positive specific granules at the electron microscope), isolated (a single affected member in each family examined), and stable (persistent at long-term follow-up) [44-45]. However, the myeloperoxidase deficiency in eosinophil is less common than neutrophil. Eosinophilic peroxidase deficiency was not correlatable with any particular disease, although a nonsignificant association with allergic-type conditions was observed [44-45]. Impairment in immune response to the parasitic infection is still controversy.

C. Basophil Enzymatic Deficiency

Basophil enzymatic deficiency is extremely rare and has never been reported in the neonate.

D. Monocyte Enzymatic Deficiency

Basically, macrophage function is insufficient if the generation of a respiratory burst is altered like in hereditary chronic granulomatous disease on one hand, but on the other hand is as well disturbed, if there is a lack in antioxidant enzyme activity [46]. Similar to neutrophil, monocyte myeloperoxidase deficiency can be seen. The patients with monocyte myleoperoxidase deficiency can present frequent infections due to the impairment of phagocytosis mechanism. Myeloperoxisase deficiency associated with severe sepsis is rarely reported [47].

E. Lymphocyte Enzymatic Deficiency

Lymphocyte enzymatic deficiency is not common but immunodeficiency due to the defect of lymphocyte cell is common. The details on the congenital lymphocyte – related immune deficiency can be seen in another chapter in this book. The well-known example of rare lymphocyte enzymatic deficiencies is adenosine deaminase deficiency. Genetic deficiencies in the purine catabolic enzyme adenosine deaminase in humans results primarily in a severe lymphopenia and immunodeficiency that can lead to the death of affected individuals early in life [48]. The metabolic basis of the immunodeficiency is likely related to the sensitivity of lymphocytes to the accumulation of the adenosine deaminase substrates adenosine and 2'-deoxyadenosine [48]. Deficiency of adenosine deaminase results in severe combined immunodeficiency [48-49]. Clinical cure has been observed in several adenosine deaminase -severe combined immunodeficiency patients after bone marrow transplantation in which only donor T cells were engrafted, suggesting that T-cell correction alone is sufficient for full immune reconstitution [49]. Children without an HLA-matched donor have been treated with polyethylene glycol- adenosine deaminase as enzyme replacement therapy, resulting in varying degrees of immunologic and clinical improvement [49]. A gene therapy protocol targeting peripheral blood lymphocytes (PBLs) published in 1995 is the new hope for treatment of this disorder [50-51]. Alternative therapeutic options based on correction of the defective gene by retroviral gene delivery have been used to correct adenosine deaminase-deficient severe combined immunodeficiency [50-51]. A number of clinical trials have established that ex vivo gene transfer into hematopoietic progenitor cells allows effective recovery of immune defects and that gene therapy can offer a successful alternative to transplantation [50-51].

REFERENCES

[1] Mehta A, Mason PJ, Vulliamy TJ. Glucose-6-phosphate dehydrogenase deficiency. *Baillieres Best Pract Res Clin Haematol* 2000; 13:21-38.

[2] Kaplan M, Hammerman C. Glucose-6-phosphate dehydrogenase deficiency: a potential source of severe neonatal hyperbilirubinaemia and kernicterus. *Semin Neonatol* 2002; 7:121-8.

[3] Evdokimova AI, Ryneiskaia VA, Plakhuta TG. Hemostatic changes in hereditary hemolytic anemias in children. *Pediatriia.* 1979; 8:17-21.

[4] Fujii H. Glucose-6-phosphate dehydrogenase. *Nippon Rinsho* 1995; 53:1221-5.

[5] Beutler E. G6PD: population genetics and clinical manifestations. *Blood Rev* 1996; 10:45-52.

[6] Beutler E. Study of glucose-6-phosphate dehydrogenase: history and molecular biology. *Am J Hematol* 1993; 42:53-8.

[7] Oliveira S, Pinheiro S, Gomes P, Horta AB, Castro AS. Favism. *Acta Med Port* 20001;13:237-40.

[8] Holm B, Jensenius M. Favism. Acute hemolysis after intake of fava beans. *Tidsskr Nor Laegeforen* 1998; 118:384-5.

[9] Mareni C, Repetto L, Forteleoni G, Meloni T, Gaetani GF. Favism: looking for an autosomal gene associated with glucose-6-phosphate dehydrogenase deficiency. *J Med Genet* 1984; 21:278-80.

[10] Kitayaporn D, Charoenlarp P, Pattaraarechachai J, Pholpoti T. G6PD deficiency and fava bean consumption do not produce hemolysis in Thailand. *Southeast Asian J Trop Med Public Health* 1991; 22:176-82.

[11] Damonte G, Guida L, Sdraffa A, Benatti U, Melloni E, Forteleoni G, Meloni T, Carafoli E, De Flora A. Mechanisms of perturbation of erythrocyte calcium homeostasis in favism. *Cell Calcium* 1992; 13:649-58.

[12] Kaplan M, Hammerman C. Glucose-6-phosphate dehydrogenase deficiency: a hidden risk for kernicterus. *Semin Perinatol*. 2004 Oct;28(5):356-64.

[13] Wiwanitkit V. Neonatal jaundice in glucose-6-phosphate dehydrogenase deficiency cases in different regions of Thailand. *Haema* 2005; 8(4): 713-714

[14] Corchia C, Balata A, Meloni GF, Meloni T.Favism in a female newborn infant whose mother ingested fava beans before delivery. *J Pediatr*. 1995 Nov;127(5):807-8.

[15] Chuu WM, Lin DT, Lin KH, Chen BW, Chen RL, Lin KS. Can severe neonatal jaundice be prevented by neonatal screening for glucose-6-phosphate dehydrogenase deficiency?--a review of evidence. *Zhonghua Min Guo Xiao Er Ke Yi Xue Hui Za Zhi* 1996; 37:333-41.

[16] Wiwanitkit V. Laboratory investigation in neonatal jaundice. *Med J Ubon Hosp* 2001; 22: 231-239.

[17] Pao M, Kulkarni A, Gupta V, Kaul S, Balan S. Neonatal screening for glucose-6-phosphate dehydrogenase deficiency. *Indian J Pediatr*. 2005 Oct;72(10):835-7.

[18] Brewer GJ, Tarlov AR, Alving AS. Methemoglobin reduction test - a new, simple in vitro test for identifying primaquine sensitivity. *Bull World Health Organ* 1960; 22: 633 – 40.

[19] Sanpavat S, Nuchprayoon I, Kittikalayawong A, Ungbumnet W. The value of methemoglobin reduction test as a screening test for neonatal glucose 6-phosphate dehydrogenase deficiency. *J Med Assoc Thai*. 2001; 84 Suppl 1:S91-8.

[20] Wiwanitkit V. Is the G-6-PD activity assay more cost effective than the methaemoglobin reduction test in screening for G-6-PD deficiency? *Haema* 2005; 8(1): 61-63.

[21] Corbucci GG. The role of reduced glutathione during the course of acute haemolysis in glucose-6-phosphate dehydrogenase deficient patients: clinical and pharmacodynamic aspects. *Int J Clin Pharmacol Res* 1990; 10:305-10.

[22] Tabbara IA. Hemolytic anemias. Diagnosis and management. *Med Clin North Am* 1992; 76:649-68.

[23] Zanella A, Colombo MB, Rossi F, Merati G, Sirchia G. Congenital non-spherocytic haemolytic anaemias. *Haematologica*. 1989 Jul-Aug;74(4):387-96.

[24] Zanella A, Fermo E, Bianchi P, Valentini G. Red cell pyruvate kinase deficiency: molecular and clinical aspects. *Br J Haematol*. 2005 Jul;130(1):11-25.

[25] Omine M. Hereditary hemolytic anemia due to abnormal enzymes of the glycolytic pathway. *Nippon Rinsho*. 1996 Sep;54(9):2460-6.

[26] Kanno H. Pyruvate kinase (PK) isozyme switching and genetic heterogeneity of PK deficiency. *Nippon Rinsho.* 1995 May;53(5):1213-20.

[27] Zanella A, Bianchi P. Red cell pyruvate kinase deficiency: from genetics to clinical manifestations. *Baillieres Best Pract Res Clin Haematol.* 2000 Mar;13(1):57-81.

[28] Hammer SG, Lewan RB. Neonatal hyperbilirubinemia caused by pyruvate kinase deficiency. *J Am Board Fam Pract.* 1988 Oct-Dec;1(4):288-90.

[29] Ferreira P, Morais L, Costa R, Resende C, Dias CP, Araujo F, Costa E, Barbot J, Vilarinho A. Hydrops fetalis associated with erythrocyte pyruvate kinase deficiency. *Eur J Pediatr.* 2000 Jul;159(7):481-2.

[30] Zanella A, Fermo E, Bianchi P, Chiarelli LR, Valentini G. Pyruvate kinase deficiency: The genotype-phenotype association. *Blood Rev.* 2007 Mar 12;

[31] Afriat R, Lecolier B, Prehu MO, Sauvanet E, Bercau G, Audit I, Galacteros F. Prenatal diagnosis of homozygous pyruvate kinase deficiency. *J Gynecol Obstet Biol Reprod (Paris).* 1995; 24(1):81-4.

[32] Baronciani L, Beutler E. Prenatal diagnosis of pyruvate kinase deficiency. *Blood.* 1994 Oct 1;84(7):2354-6.

[33] Kanno H. Hexokinase: gene structure and mutations. *Baillieres Best Pract Res Clin Haematol.* 2000 Mar;13(1):83-8.

[34] Murakami K, Kanno H, Tancabelic J, Fujii H. Gene expression and biological significance of hexokinase in erythroid cells. *Acta Haematol.* 2002; 108(4):204-9.

[35] Bethenod M, Kissin C, Mathieu M, Nivelon JL, Cotte J. Hexokinase deficiency of erythrocytes. Familial study of a case of primary isolated deficiency and ancassociated case with glucose-6 phosphate dehydrogenase deficiency. *Ann Pediatr (Paris).* 1967 Dec 2;14(12):826-8.

[36] Travis SF.Red cell enzymopathies in the newborn. II. Inherited deficiencies of red cell enzymes. *Ann Clin Lab Sci.* 1982 May-Jun;12(3):163-77.

[37] Shinozaki K, Komiyama A. Neutrophil pyruvate kinase deficiency. *Ryoikibetsu Shokogun Shirizu.* 2000;(32):177-8

[38] Burge PS, Johnson WS, Hayward AR. Neutrophil pyruvate kinase deficiency with recurrent staphylococcal infections: first reported case. *Br Med J.* 1976 Mar 27;1(6012):742-5.

[39] Shiohara M, Komiyama A. Myeloperoxidase deficiency. *Ryoikibetsu Shokogun Shirizu.* 2000; (32):183-5.

[40] Lanfa F. Clinical manifestation of myeloperoxidase deficiency. *J Mol Med.* 1998 Sep;76(10):676-81.

[41] Nauseef WM. Insights into myeloperoxidase biosynthesis from its inherited deficiency. *J Mol Med.* 1998 Sep;76(10):661-8.

[42] Baehner RL. Neutrophil dysfunction associated with states of chronic and recurrent infection. *Pediatr Clin North Am.* 1980 May;27(2):377-401.

[43] Rider ED, Christensen RD, Hall DC, Rothstein G. Myeloperoxidase deficiency in neutrophils of neonates. *J Pediatr.* 1988 Apr;112(4):648-51.

[44] Kutter D, Mueller-Hagedorn S, Forges T, Glaesener R. A case of eosinophil peroxidase deficiency. *Ann Hematol.* 1995 Dec;71(6):315-7.

[45] Cappelletti P, Doretto P, Signori D, Bizzaro N. Eosinophilic peroxidase deficiency. Cytochemical and ultrastructural characterization of 21 new cases. *Am J Clin Pathol.* 1992 Dec;98(6):615-22.

[46] Ebert-Dumig R, Seufert J, Schneider D, Kohrle J, Schutze N, Jakob F. Expression of selenoproteins in monocytes and macrophages--implications for the immune system. *Med Klin (Munich)*. 1999 Oct 15;94 Suppl 3:29-34.

[47] Grossl NA, Candel AG, Shrit A, Schumacher HR. Myeloperoxidase deficiency and severe sepsis. *South Med J.* 1993 Jul;86(7):832-6.

[48] Blackburn MR, Kellems RE. Adenosine deaminase deficiency: metabolic basis of immune deficiency and pulmonary inflammation. *Adv Immunol.* 2005; 86:1-41.

[49] Blaese RM. Development of gene therapy for immunodeficiency: adenosine deaminase deficiency. *Pediatr Res*. 1993 Jan;33(1 Suppl):S49-53.

[50] Sakiyama Y, Ariga T, Ohtsu M. Gene therapy for adenosine deaminase deficiency. *Nippon Rinsho*. 2005 Mar;63(3):448-52.

[51] Gaspar HB, Thrasher AJ. Gene therapy for severe combined immunodeficiencies. *Expert Opin Biol Ther*. 2005 Sep;5(9):1175-82.

Chapter 11

PORPHYRIA

INTRODUCTION

Porphyria is a compelling disease with disrupted enzyme pathways, heightened sensitivities, and a fascinating history tied in with tales of Dracula [1]. The porphyrias comprise a clinically and genetically heterogeneous group of diseases mostly arising from a genetically determined dysfunction of specific enzymes along the pathway of heme biosynthesis [2]. Based on the occurrence or absence of cutaneous symptoms and life-threatening acute neurological attacks, the different types of porphyrias can either be classified into cutaneous and non-cutaneous forms or acute and non-acute forms [2]. Since besides the skin, other organs can be affected, such as the liver and the central nervous system, therefore, interdisciplinary supervision of these patients is mandatory [3]. Establishing an accurate diagnosis might be difficult for two reasons: i) the porphyrias can manifest with a broad but unspecific spectrum of clinical symptoms mimicking several other disorders, and ii) biochemical examination of urine, feces, and blood can reveal overlapping findings [2]. Recent advances in the molecular understanding of the porphyrias now offer specific diagnosis and precise definition of the types of genetic mutations involved in the disease [4]. Molecular diagnostic testing is powerful and very useful in kindred evaluation and genetic counseling when a disease-responsible mutation has been identified in the family. It is also the only way to properly screen asymptomatic gene carriers, facilitating correct treatment and appropriate genetic counseling of family members at risk [4]. In this chapter, the clinical information on porphyria will be summarized.

HEME BIOSYNTHESIS PATHWAY

Heme is a complex of iron with protoporphyrin IX that is essential for the function of all aerobic cells [5]. Heme serves as the prosthetic group of numerous hemoproteins (including hemoglobin, myoglobin, cytochromes, guanylate cyclase, and nitric oxide synthase) and plays an important role in controlling protein synthesis and cell differentiation [5]. There are eight enzymes in the heme biosynthetic pathway and three enzymes in the heme catabolic pathway. Enzymatic defects in heme biosynthesis lead to clinical conditions termed porphyrias.

Cellular heme levels are tightly controlled; this is achieved by a fine balance between heme biosynthesis and catabolism by the enzyme heme oxygenase [5]. Most iron in mammalian systems is routed to mitochondria to serve as a substrate for ferrochelatase [6]. Basically, ferrochelatase (E.C. 4.99.1.1) is a homodimeric (86 kDa) molecule [7-8]. The enzyme contains two NO-sensitive and uniquely coordinated [2Fe-2S] clusters [8]. Its membrane association is mediated in part by a 12-residue hydrophobic lip that also forms the entrance to the active site pocket [8]. Physiologically, ferrochelatase inserts iron into protoporphyrin IX to form heme which is incorporated into hemoglobin and cytochromes, the dominant hemoproteins in mammals [6]. The recently solved x-ray structure of human ferrochelatase identifies a potential binding site for an iron donor protein on the matrix side of the homodimer [7]. Yoon and Cowan demonstrated Hs holofrataxin to be a high affinity iron binding partner for Hs ferrochelatase that is capable of both delivering iron to ferrochelatase and mediating the terminal step in mitochondrial heme biosynthesis [7]. According to this study, a general regulatory mechanism for mitochondrial iron metabolism is described that defines frataxin involvement in both heme and iron-sulfur cluster biosyntheses [7]. At present, the complete DNA sequences of 45 ferrochelatases from procaryotes and eucaryotes are available [9]. These sequences along with direct protein studies reveal that ferrochelatases, while related, vary significantly in amino acid sequence, molecular size, subunit composition, solubility, and the presence or absence of nitric-oxide-sensitive [2Fe-2S] cluster [9].

Tissue-specific regulatory features characterize the heme biosynthetic pathway [6]. Ponka and Schulman proposed that that iron metabolism and heme synthesis were controlled by distinct mechanisms in erythroid versus nonerythroid cells [10]. In erythroid cells, regulation is mediated by erythroid-specific transcription factors and the availability of iron as Fe/S clusters [6]. Differences in iron metabolism and in genes for 5-aminolevulinic acid synthase (ALA-S, the first enzyme in heme biosynthesis) are responsible for the differences in regulation and rates of heme synthesis in erythroid and nonerythroid cells [5]. There are 2 different genes for ALA-S, one of which is expressed ubiquitously (ALA-S1), whereas the expression of the other (ALA-S2) is specific to erythroid cells [5]. On a per-cell basis, the rate of heme synthesis in the developing erythroid cells is at least 1 order of magnitude higher than in the liver, which is in turn the second most active heme producer in the organism [5]. In non-erythroid cells the pathway is regulated by heme-mediated feedback inhibition [6]. However, at least two enzymes exist as isozymes between erythroid and non-erythroid tissues [11]. One is ALA-S, and the erythroid and hepatic isozymes are coded by two separate genes [11]. The other is porphobilinogen deaminase (PBGD), and both the erythroid and the non-erythroid PBGD mRNA are transcribed from a single PBGD gene by alternate transcription and splicing [11].

History of Porphyria

Prophyria is a disorder with a long history. The first iconographic description of hepatoerythropoietic porphyria was described in 1599. The subject drawn by physician Aldrovandi is a 20-year-old girl showing remarkable facial hypertrichosis, while her body is described as hairless [12]. It was also proposed that the episodic madness suffered by King George III (1738-1820) resulted from an acute hereditary porphyria, variegate porphyria, caused by deficiency of protoporphyrinogen oxidase [13-14]. The diagnosis was based on the historical archive and a contentious claim that living members of the House of Hanover were affected with the condition [13]. A re-examination of the medical evidence and the appearance of new historical material have suggested that porphyria did indeed exist in the Royal Houses of Europe[13]. Acute intermittent porphyria is also a possible illness of the famous world musician, Vincent van Gogh [15]. Indeed, the pophyria might be older than 16th century. Dracula or vampire in the old belief might be a description of porphyria. Key clinical features of the horror movie vampires illustrate a variety of pearls in the diagnosis of a variety of neurological disorders, including porphyria [16].

Clinical Presentation of Porphyria

Clinically, porphyria is a group of inherited disorders of heme biosynthesis clinically classified as neurovisceral, cutaneous, or mixed. Porphyrias can be classified as either hepatic or erythroid, depending on the major production site of porphyrins or their precursors. Porphyria is often misdiagnosed because patients have vague symptoms. However, acute forms of porphyria can be life-threatening, so it is important to make an accurate diagnosis and initiate proper management. Medically, acute porphyria is a disorder caused by a change in the amount of porphyrins (nitrogen-containing substances) found in the blood, resulting in acute abdominal pain, skin lesions, light sensitivity, anemia, and neurological changes.

A. Acute Intermittent Porphyria

Acute intermittent porphyria (AIP) is one of the porphyriaswhihc manifests itself by abdomen pain, neuropathies, and constipation, but, unlike most types of porphyria, patients with AIP do not have a significant cutaneous manifestation. It is an autosomal dominant condition with incomplete penetrance and is potentially life-threatening [17]. The disease is caused by a partial deficiency of porphobilinogen deaminase (PBGD), also called hydroxymethyl bilane synthase, in heme biosynthesis [18]. The prevalence of AIP varies geographically. The common clinical pattern of symptom involves acute abdominal pain, psychiatric disturbances, and acute neuropathy [19]. Clinical diagnosis is not difficult when doctors keep the possibility of AIP in their minds in cases of abdominal pain, weakness and mental symptoms [19]. These symptoms occur during acute attacks, which are often precipitated by drugs, alcohol, low caloric intake, or infections [20]. The key point in management is to suspect and confirm the diagnosis as early as possible in order to treat the attack and to avoid inappropriate treatments which may exacerbate the crisis [17]. Although the pathophysiology of the disease has not yet been fully elucidated, a specific treatment of acute attacks with heme has improved the prognosis [20]. Measurement of urinary PBG is the best biochemical test for AIP, although it is unspecific and does not distinguish AIP from other acute porphyrias [21]. Since biochemical measurements of patients and their healthy relatives overlap, the diagnosis of AIP may remain undetermined at the symptom-free phase [18]. Because the acute increase in PBG is often modest, the medical history, signs, and symptoms must be evaluated carefully during an acute attack [21]. The high prevalence of acute intermittent porphyria in specific geographic areas emphasizes the importance of correct diagnosis, the first crucial step in avoiding attacks and associated diseases [22]. Mutation detection in AIP, which provides 95% sensitivity and around 100% specificity, has quickly been incorporated into good clinical practice [18]. The nerve biopsy usually shows segmental demyelination and axonal degeneration [19]. Many small vacuolations are distinctively seen in all of the cell components of the nerve [19].

B. Porphyria Cutanea Tarda

Corphyria cutanea tarda (PCT) is a term encompassing a group of disorders in which activity of the heme synthetic enzyme uroporphyrinogen decarboxylase (UROD) is deficient. PCT is the commonest of all porphyrias and usually characterized by blisters and fragility of skin in light-exposed areas [23]. Excess porphyrins in the skin interact with light of approximately 400 nm-wavelength radiant energy, forming reactive oxygen species [24]. It can be clinically indistinguishable from other disorders including variegate porphyria and the diagnosis can only be made by rigorous biochemical analysis [23]. It is usually an acquired condition caused by inhibition of the uroporphyrinogen decarboxylase enzyme in the liver [23]. Hereditary haemochromatosis, hepatitis C virus infection, alcohol, oestrogens and a family history of PCT are the major risk factors for the condition and should be searched for specifically in all patients [23]. PCT also includes familial types with *UROD* gene mutations and acquired types that may occur in individuals with a genetic predisposition (sporadic PCT) after exposure to hepatotoxins or in the context of hepatic tumors. In addition, porphyria cutanea tarda is associated with an increased incidence of the haemochromatosis gene [24]. PCT may also follow exposure to porphyrogenic toxic chemicals [25]. Clinically overt PCT (types I and II) is provoked by liver cell injury, particularly when associated with alcohol abuse, hepatitis C infection, or estrogens [25]. Hemochromatosis has a significant clinical correlation to PCT. Hepatic iron overload is common, depletion of iron stores produces remission, and their replenishment leads to relapse [25]. Iron, by catalyzing the formation of reactive oxygen species, can enhance uroporphyrin formation by increasing the rate at which uroporphyrinogen is oxidized to urophophyrin [26]. Iron may also act indirectly to inhibit uroporphyrinogen decarboxylase activity by enhancing the formation of non-porphyrin products of porphyrinogen oxidation that are themselves direct inhibitors of the enzyme [26]. Finally, iron can act to increase urophorphyrin production by inducing delta-aminolevulinic acid synthase, thus increasing the amount of delta-aminolevulinic acid, the precursor to uroporphyrinogen, present in the cell [26]. For PCT, coral pink fluorescence of uroporphyrins in an acidified urine specimen is diagnostic [27-28].Treatments for PCT include withdrawal of aggravating factors, phlebotomy and oral antimalarial medications [24]. Therapeutic venesection reduces the iron load and the uroporphyrins are mobilized by treatment with hydroxychloroquine [27]. An increased risk of liver cirrhosis and hepatocellular carcinoma may presumably be reduced by early diagnosis and treatment [27].

DIAGNOSIS OF PORPHYRIA

A. Diagnosis of Acute Porphyria

Concerning porphyria, a deficiency of any of the 8 enzymes in the biosynthetic pathway can lead to a variety of clinical symptoms. Classification depends on the defective enzyme5. Molecularly, Martinez di Montemuros et al performed a study in Italy and identified 50 different mutations among 4 genes associated with the most common porphyrias showing a high molecular heterogeneity: 22 in the hydroxymethylbilane synthetase (HMBS) gene (AIP), 7 in the protoporphyrinogen oxidase (PPOX) gene (VP), 16 in the uroporphyrinogen decarboxylase (UROD) gene (PCT) and 5 in the ferrochelatase (FECH) gene (EPP) [29]. For definitive diagnosis, the only acceptable method of porphyrin diagnosis is by porphyrin quantitation using high-performance liquid chromatograpy or thinlayer chromatography coupled with fluorometric detection and quantitation [30]. Equalitative methods and solvent extraction are not acceptable. Negative, doubtful and low-level positive results are unacceptable and must be followed by chromatographic confirmation. However, in acute porphyria which is an emergencyin laboratory medicine, an effective screening test is required. In those cases, performing an urgent Watson- Schwartz reaction with Ehrlich.s aldehyde, and follow up with quantitation of ALA and PBG. Thereafter confirm the type of porphyria present by either biochemical porphyrin quantitation, or by a R59W test followed by porphyrin quantitation if R59W negative is recommended [30-32].

Ehrlich.s reagent, also known as Ehrlich.s diazo reagent is a well know reagent first produced by Paul Ehrlich. This reagent is widely used for first diagnosis of acute porphyria. The composition is 2 g% p-dimethyl aminobenzaldehyde in 20%-ig HCI [33]. The major test using this reagent is Ehrlich.s aldehyde test, which is used to perform an emergent diagnosis of acute intermittent porphyria [33]. For performing the test, equal volumes of urine and Ehrlich.s reagent are mixed [33]. If a pink colour is formed this indicates a raised urinary concentration of either porphobilinogen or urobilinogen [33]. In cases of raised porphobilinogen, as in acute intermittent porphyria, the pink precipitate is observed to be insoluble in chloroform [33]. The other usage of this reagent is in histopathology. After some modification of Ehrlich.s reagent, the formaldehyde-Schiff.s reagent can be derived [33]. The use of formaldehyde-Schiff.s reagent as a nucleolar stain has been widely used [34]. Using different digestion procedures, it was confirmed that the stain is specific for RNA. In addition, it can be suitably used as a nucleolar stain, particularly in plant materials after a short TCA extraction, which probably extracts the nonbound RNA [34].

However, it is somtimes difficult to suspect the diagnosis of acute porphyria in real medical practice. There is a very characteristic discrepancy between the serious complaints and the actual clinical findings [35]. The severe cramping abdominal pain, nausea, vomiting, muscle weakness of the limbs and sensory loss are the main signs at the beginning [35]. The specific symptoms which help to establish the diagnosis--red-colored urine, hyponatremia, tachycardia, hypertension, subileus, acute psychosis, gradually developing paresis of the lower and then the upper limbs--are characteristic for the later phase of the acute attack [35]. Very often there is a rapid progression with Landry-type paralysis developing in days or even in hours, following respiratory paralysis or serious arrhythmia is the cause of the death [35]. Sies et al proposed that porphyria might present (1) with acute symptoms, which may be abdominal pain, neurological or psychiatric; (2) with skin rash or photosensitivity; or (3) with a putative family history [36]. The recognition of the overt disorder with extrahepatic manifestations depends on the demonstration of biochemical abnormalities due to these primary defects and compensatory hepatic overexpression of hepatic delta-aminolaevulinic acid synthase in the acute porphyrias [37]. Consequently, haem precursors are synthesized in excess [37]. The increased metabolites upstream of the enzymatic defect are excreted into urine and faeces and the diagnosis is based on their evaluation [37]. Sies et al also proposed that screening for latent porphyria has been greatly facilitated by fluorescence emission scanning of plasma and by mutational analysis [36]. Thunell et al said that early diagnosis was of prime importance since it made way for counseling with the aim to block the development of acute, as well as late, disease [38]. They said that the strain imposed upon the diagnostic process made management in specialized laboratories necessary [38]. Inadvertent handling of the diagnostic procedures in laboratories lacking in knowledge, experience and technical competence is repeatedly the reason for harmful underdiagnosis and overdiagnosis [38]. Thunell et al concluded that gene diagnosis of the carrier condition, principally within reach in all types of acute porphyria, was of incomparable versatility and accuracy [38].

B. Diagnosis of Porphyria Cutanea Tarda

Deficiency of the fifth enzyme in haem synthesis, UPGD, known as PCT may give rise to accumulation and excretion of poly-carboxylated porphyrins, as well as to clinical manifestations in the form of a phototoxic skin reaction and liver engagement leading to cirrhosis and hepatocellular cancer. Dominant clinical symptoms are bullae, increased cutaneous vulnerability, hypertrichosis and elastosis [39]. Biochemically, total porphyrin levels in urine are increased with a predominance of uroporphyrin and heptacarboxylic porphyrin. Isocoproporphyrin is demonstrable in feces [39]. Campo et al also proposed that the finding in a liver biopsy specimen of hemosiderin in periportal hepatocytes, fatty changes and portal inflammation should alert one to the possible diagnosis of PCT [40].

C. Screening for Porphyria in Newborn

Porphyria in childhood is an uncommon problem but the recognition of these disorders is vitally important for affected children [41-42]. Of the cutaneous porphyrias, erythropoietic protoporphyria, congenital erythropoietic porphyria, hepatoerythropoietic porphyria, and the hereditary form of porphyria cutanea tarda (PCT) can present in infancy or childhood [41-42]. Screening for porphyria in newborn is an important primary prevention for porphyria [43-44]. However, it has not been yet included as a routine screening program.

TREATMENT FOR PORPHYRIA

A. Treatment for acute porphyria

Although mild attacks sometimes respond to glucose administration, severe attacks or symptoms that are likely to progress should be treated with heme. Heme preparations are now available for the specific treatment of attacks of acute porphyria [45]. Specific treatment with heme preparations should be instituted as soon as possible following confirmation of increased excretion of porphobilinogen in the urine [46]. The heme arginate (dose of 250 mg or 3 mg/kg, start within 24 hours) and hematin are the two widely used heme preparation for facing up with an acute porphyria attack [47]. Heme arginate is more preferable to hematin in the treatment of acute porphyrias because of its better stability, fewer side effects, and better documentation of its benefits [48]. Favorable responses in attack can be derived by heme arginate [47]. The only side effect is moderate thrombophlebitis in only a few patients [48]. The prognosis of acute attacks has been greatly improved since the introduction of heme-arginate in the 1980's [49]. Supportive treatment includes opiate analgesia, monitoring for and treating complications such as hypertension and hyponatraemia [46]. Follow-up should include counseling on lifestyle modification involving avoidance of alcohol, smoking and known porphyrogenic drugs and diet [46]. Identification and counseling of at risk relatives is essential [46].

B. Treatment for porphyria cutanea tarda

The basis of treatment of PCT consists of three elements: avoidance of triggering factors, skin care, iron depletion and porphyrin elimination [50]. Alcohol and certain systemic medical drugs, such as oestrogens (or tuberculostatics), should be considered as triggering factors, and as far as possible, avoided [50]. Other triggering factors, such as chronic haemodialysis in renal insufficiency, need a different approach. The hallmark in iron depletion is phlebotomy [50]. PCT can be effectively treated by phlebotomy or low dose chloroquine [46]. Best therapeutic strategies are the oral administration of chloroquine 125 mg twice a week and repetitive bloodlettings or the combination of both. To date, HIV-seropositive cases with PCT can also be seen. A possible correlation between HIV and PCT has been proposed for a few years but there is no specific explanation [51]. Similar to non-HIV infected patients, successful therapeutic approaches for PCT in the patients with HIV infection included (a) elimination of PCT-precipitating agents, (b) avoidance of sun exposure, and (c) periodic phlebotomy [52].

C. Treatment for congenital porphyria

Congenital erythropoietic porphyria (CEP, Gunther's disease) is an extremely rare autosomal recessive disease, characterized by mutilating cutaneous photosensitivity and abnormal haem synthesis in the bone marrow [53]. Reduced activity of uroporphyrinogen III synthase (UROIIIS), the fourth enzyme of haem biosynthetic pathway causes this disease [53]. The consequences of chronic haemolysis are splenomegaly, reactive erythroid hyperplasia, erythrodontia, bone fragility, extreme photosensitivity and photomutilation [54]. Congenital erythropoietic porphyria is a rare, early onset, severe, photomutilating condition for which bone marrow transplantation has been shown to be successful [46]. If patients with this disease have an HLA-matched sibling, then stem cell transplantation should be strongly considered because this is currently the only known curative therapy [55-56]. The new concept for treatment of congenital porphyria is gene therapy. Tehre are several attempts to develop new gene therapy method for congenital porphyria. Recently, Mazurier et al investigated retroviral transfer in deficient human fibroblasts, immortalized lymphoblasts as well as bone marrow cells, and obtained a complete restoration of the enzymatic activity and full metabolic correction [57]. The future availability of a mouse model of the disease will permit ex vivo gene therapy experiments on the entire animal [57-58].

PSUEDOPORPHYRIA

Pseudoporphyria is the term used to describe a photodistributed bullous disorder with clinical and histologic features of porphyria cutanea tarda, but without accompanying biochemical porphyrin abnormalities [59]. Medications, chronic renal failure/dialysis, excessive sun exposure and UVA radiation have all been reported to cause pseudoporphyria [59]. Pseudoporphyria might mimic the cutaneous symptoms of PCT in the setting of normal or near-normal porphyrin levels in the serum, urine, or stool [60]. Despite efforts to discontinue an offending medication, symptoms may persist indefinitely [60]. Schanbacher et al studied 20 cases of psuedophilia. According to their study, the major presenting clinical features were blistering, scarring, photosensitivity, skin fragility, and milia [60]. Histologically, most patients had classic findings of subepidermal separation with festooning of dermal papillae [60]. Most cases of pseudoporphyria are drug-induced. Naproxen, the most common offender, has been associated with a dimorphic clinical pattern: a PCT-like presentation and one simulating erythropoietic protoporphyria in the pediatric population [61]. Other NSAIDs of the propionic acid family can also cause pseudoporphyria [61]. Hemodialysis-associated pseudoporphyria is also reported. It is successfully responding to treatment with oral N-acetylcysteine [62]. Antioxidant properties of oral N-acetylcysteine are believed to be an important underlying for treatment of hemodialysis-associated pseudoporphyria [62].

REFERENCES

[1] Norman RA. Past and future: porphyria and porphyrins. *Skinmed.* 2005 Sep-Oct;4(5):287-92.

[2] Poblete-Gutierrez P, Wiederholt T, Merk HF, Frank J. The porphyrias: clinical presentation, diagnosis and treatment. *Eur J Dermatol.* 2006 May-Jun;16(3):230-40.

[3] Poblete-Gutierrez P, Wiederholt T, Merk HF, Frank J. Laboratory tests and therapeutic strategies for the porphyrias. *Hautarzt.* 2006 May 3;

[4] Sassa S. Modern diagnosis and management of the porphyrias. *Br J Haematol.* 2006 Nov;135(3):281-92.

[5] Ponka P. Cell biology of heme. *Am J Med Sci.* 1999 Oct;318(4):241-56.

[6] Ajioka RS, Phillips JD, Kushner JP. Biosynthesis of heme in mammals. *Biochim Biophys Acta.* 2006 Jul;1763(7):723-36.

[7] Frataxin-mediated iron delivery to ferrochelatase in the final step of heme biosynthesis. *J Biol Chem.* 2004 Jun 18;279(25):25943-6.

[8] Wu CK, Dailey HA, Rose JP, Burden A, Sellers VM, Wang BC. The enzyme contains two NO-sensitive and uniquely coordinated [2Fe-2S] clusters. Its membrane association is mediated in part by a 12-residue hydrophobic lip that also forms the entrance to the active site pocket. *Nat Struct Biol.* 2001 Feb;8(2):156-60.

[9] Dailey HA, Dailey TA, Wu CK, Medlock AE, Wang KF, Rose JP, Wang BC. Ferrochelatase at the millennium: structures, mechanisms and [2Fe-2S] clusters. *Cell Mol Life Sci.* 2000 Dec;57(13-14):1909-26.

[10]Ponka P, Schulman HM. Regulation of heme biosynthesis: distinct regulatory features in erythroid cells. *Stem Cells.* 1993 May;11 Suppl 1:24-35.

[11]Sassa S. Regulation of the genes for heme pathway enzymes in erythroid and in non-erythroid cells. *Int J Cell Cloning.* 1990 Jan;8(1):10-26.

[12]Biolcati G, Dolazza C. 1599: first iconographic description of hepatoerythropoietic porphyria. *Int J Dermatol.* 2006 Aug;45(8):976-8.

[13]Cox TM, Jack N, Lofthouse S, Watling J, Haines J, Warren MJ. Pascuzzi RM. King George III and porphyria: an elemental hypothesis and investigation. *Lancet.* 2005 Jul 23-29;366(9482):332-5.

[14]Croarkin P. From King George to neuroglobin: the psychiatric aspects of acute intermittent porphyria. *J Psychiatr Pract.* 2002 Nov;8(6):398-405.

[15]Hughes JR. A reappraisal of the possible seizures of Vincent van Gogh. *Epilepsy Behav.* 2005 Jun;6(4):504-10.

[16]Pascuzzi RM. Pearls and pitfalls in the horror cinema. *Semin Neurol.* 1998;18(2):267-73.

[17]Herrick AL, McColl KE. Acute intermittent porphyria. *Best Pract Res Clin Gastroenterol.* 2005;19:235-49.

[18]Kauppinen R. Molecular diagnostics of acute intermittent porphyria. *Expert Rev Mol Diagn.* 2004 Mar;4(2):243-9.

[19]Sugimura K. Acute intermittent porphyria. *Nippon Rinsho.* 1995 Jun;53(6):1418-21.

[20]Grandchamp B. Acute intermittent porphyria. *Semin Liver Dis.* 1998;18(1):17-24.

[21]Kauppinen R, von und zu Fraunberg M. Molecular and biochemical studies of acute intermittent porphyria in 196 patients and their families. *Clin Chem.* 2002 Nov;48(11):1891-900.

[22]Tollali G, Nielsen EW, Brekke OL. Acute intermittent porphyria. *Tidsskr Nor Laegeforen.* 2002;122:1102-5.

[23]Sarkany RP. The management of porphyria cutanea tarda. *Clin Exp Dermatol.* 2001 May;26(3):225-32.

[24]Bleasel NR, Varigos GA. Porphyria cutanea tarda. *Australas J Dermatol.* 2000 Nov;41(4):197-206

[25]Elder GH. Porphyria cutanea tarda. *Semin Liver Dis.* 1998;18(1):67-75.

[26]Lambrecht RW, Bonkovsky HL. Hemochromatosis and porphyria. *Semin Gastrointest Dis.* 2002 Apr;13(2):109-19.

[27]Bygum A, Brandrup F, Christiansen L, Petersen NE. Porphyria cutanea tarda. *Ugeskr Laeger.* 2000 Apr 3;162(14):2020-4.

[28]Khoo BP, Tay YK. Porphyria cutanea tarda. *Singapore Med J.* 2000 Jun;41(6):292-4.

[29]Martinez di Montemuros F, Di Pierro E, Patti E, Tavazzi D, Danielli MG, Biolcati G, Rocchi E, Cappellini MD. Molecular characterization of porphyrias in Italy: a diagnostic flow-chart. *Cell Mol Biol (Noisy-le-grand).* 2002; 48: 867-876.

[30]Foran SE, Abel G. Guide to porphyrias. A historical and clinical perspective. *Am J Clin Pathol.* 2003; 119 (suppl): S86-S93.

[31]Tasnadi G, Bor M, Pusztai A, Szekely E. Acute porphyrias in differential diagnosis. *Orv Hetil.* 2003; 144: 811-818.

[32]Pretorius C, du Toit JJ, du Preez JC, Meissner PN. Diagnosis of variegate porphyria at birth by demonstration of the R59W mutation. *S Afr Med J.* 1997; 87: 763.

[33]Wiwanitkit V. Ehrlich reagent and diagnosis of acute porphyria: a note from Thailand. *Haema* 2004; 7(4): 463-465

[34]Ghosh S. Formaldehyde-Schiff.s reagent as a nucleolar strain. *Experientia* 1976; 32: 673-674.

[35]Tasnadi G, Bor M, Pusztai A, Szekely E. Acute porphyrias in differential diagnosis. *Orv Hetil.* 2003 Apr 27;144(17):811-8

[36]Sies C, Florkowski C, George P, Potter H. Clinical indications for the investigation of porphyria: case examples and evolving laboratory approaches to its diagnosis in New Zealand. *N Z Med J.* 2005 Sep 16;118(1222):U1658.

[37]Gross U, Hoffmann GF, Doss MO. Erythropoietic and hepatic porphyrias. *J Inherit Metab Dis.* 2000 Nov;23(7):641-61.

[38]Thunell S, Harper P, Brock A, Petersen NE. Porphyrins, porphyrin metabolism and porphyrias. II. Diagnosis and monitoring in the acute porphyrias. *Scand J Clin Lab Invest.* 2000 Nov;60(7):541-59.

[39]Fritsch C, Lang K, von Schmiedeberg S, Bolsen K, Merk H, Lehmann P, Ruzicka T. Porphyria cutanea tarda. *Skin Pharmacol Appl Skin Physiol.* 1998 Nov-Dec;11(6):321-35.

[40]Campo E, Bruguera M, Rodes J. Are there diagnostic histologic features of porphyria cutanea tarda in liver biopsy specimens? *Liver.* 1990 Jun;10(3):185-90.

[41]Jensen JD, Resnick SD. Porphyria in childhood. Semin Dermatol. 1995 Mar;14(1):33-9.

[42]Ahmed I. Childhood porphyrias. *Mayo Clin Proc.* 2002 Aug;77(8):825-36.

[43]Czartoryska B. Prenatal diagnosis: a chance? risk? dilemma? *Postepy Biochem.* 1990;36(3-4):31-3.

[44]Screening for inborn errors of metabolism. Report of a WHO Scientific Group. *World Health Organ Tech Rep Ser.* 1968;401:1-57.

[45]Elder GH, Hift RJ. Treatment of acute porphyria. *Hosp Med.* 2001 Jul;62(7):422-5.

[46]Badminton MN, Elder GH. Management of acute and cutaneous porphyrias. *Int J Clin Pract.* 2002 May;56(4):272-8.

[47]Mustajoki P, Nordmann Y. Early administration of heme arginate for acute porphyric attacks. *Arch Intern Med.* 1993 Sep 13;153(17):2004-8.

[48]Tenhunen R, Mustajoki P. Acute porphyria: treatment with heme. *Semin Liver Dis.* 1998;18(1):53-5.

[49]Nordmann Y, Deybach JC. Acute attacks of hepatic porphyria: specific treatment with heme arginate. *Ann Med Interne (Paris).* 1993;144(3):165-7.

[50]Kostler E, Wollina U. Therapy of porphyria cutanea tarda. *Expert Opin Pharmacother.* 2005 Mar;6(3):377-83.

[51]el Sayed F, Viraben R, Bazex J, Gorguet B. Porphyria cutanea tarda and HIV-1 infection. 2 new cases. *Ann Dermatol Venereol.* 1993;120(6-7):455-7.

[52]Cohen PR. Porphyria cutanea tarda in human immunodeficiency virus-seropositive men: case report and literature review. *J Acquir Immune Defic Syndr.* 1991;4(11):1112-7.

[53]Tanigawa K, Takamura N, Yamashita S. Congenital erythropoietic porphyria. *Nippon Rinsho.* 1995 Jun;53(6):1422-6.

[54]Dawe SA, Peters TJ, Du Vivier A, Creamer JD. Congenital erythropoietic porphyria: dilemmas in present day management. *Clin Exp Dermatol.* 2002 Nov;27(8):680-3.

[55]Shaw PH, Mancini AJ, McConnell JP, Brown D, Kletzel M. Treatment of congenital erythropoietic porphyria in children by allogeneic stem cell transplantation: a case report and review of the literature. *Bone Marrow Transplant.* 2001 Jan;27(1):101-5.

[56]Desnick RJ, Astrin KH. Congenital erythropoietic porphyria: advances in pathogenesis and treatment. *Br J Haematol.* 2002 Jun;117(4):779-95.

[57]Mazurier F, Moreau-Gaudry F, Salesse S, Barbot C, Ged C, Reiffers J, de Verneuil H. Gene transfer of the uroporphyrinogen III synthase cDNA into haematopoietic progenitor cells in view of a future gene therapy in congenital erythropoietic porphyria. *J Inherit Metab Dis.* 1997 Jun;20(2):247-57.

[58]de Verneuil H, Moreau-Gaudry F, Ged C. A model of congenital erythropoietic porphyria for gene transfer in hematopoietic cells. *Transfus Clin Biol.* 1997;4(3):263-6.

[59]Green JJ, Manders SM. Pseudoporphyria. *J Am Acad Dermatol.* 2001 Jan;44(1):100-8.

[60]Schanbacher CF, Vanness ER, Daoud MS, Tefferi A, Su WP. Pseudoporphyria: a clinical and biochemical study of 20 patients. *Mayo Clin Proc.* 2001 May;76(5):488-92.

[61]Al-Khenaizan S, Schechter JF, Sasseville D. Pseudoporphyria induced by propionic acid derivatives. *J Cutan Med Surg.* 1999 Jan;3(3):162-6.

[62]Cooke NS, McKenna K. A case of haemodialysis-associated pseudoporphyria successfully treated with oral N-acetylcysteine. *Clin Exp Dermatol.* 2007 Jan;32(1):64-6.

Chapter 12

NEONATAL LUPUS SYNDROME

INTRODUCTION

Systemic lupus erythrematosus (SLE) is an important autoimmune disorder. SLE is a complex polygenic autoimmune disease characterized by the presence of anti-nuclear autoantibodies (ANAs) that are often detectable years prior to the onset of clinical disease. The disease is associated with a chronic activation of the immune system, with the most severe forms progressing to inflammatory damage that can impact multiple organ systems in afflicted individuals [1]. Overactive B cells, abnormally activated T cells and inappropriate handling of cellular debris by the innate immune system are central in the pathogenesis of SLE [2]. As a model, the cases with susceptible underlying genetic factor when expose to the trigger, they will develop abnormal immune response and lead to the final immune complex induced pathology or type 3 hypersensitivity. Recent advances in molecular genetics has led to a better understanding of the genes predisposing to systemic lupus erythematosus in both humans and laboratory animal models [3]. Identification of susceptibility genes provides key insights into the pathogenesis of systemic lupus erythematosus, making new prophylactic and therapeutic approaches feasible [3]. In human lupus, case- control studies have established associations of SLE with certain major histocompatibility class II alleles, complement deficiencies, and polymorphisms of Fc gamma receptor genes, a complement-related gene, and cytokine genes [4]. Elegant genetic dissection has demonstrated that a component phenotype of SLE is displayed by each congenic strain carrying a single susceptibility locus on a resistant genetic background, whereas polycongenic strains exhibit fatal lupus nephritis [5]. During the past several years, linkage analyses using SLE multiplex families have provided many chromosomal regions for further exploration of susceptibility genes. Six regions exhibiting significant linkage to SLE are promising [4].

SLE can be seen in both sexes but it is more common in female. Children and adolescents represent 15-20% of all SLE patients [6]. Although the clinical presentation and immunological findings are similar to those of adult SLE, children usually have a more severe disease at onset with higher rates of organ involvement [6]. Rapid diagnosis and subsequent therapy are necessary to prevent major organ damage [6]. The survival of children with SLE has improved dramatically over the past decades due to the introduction of steroids and immunosuppressive drugs [6]. There is a diverse array of presenting features in childhood SLE [7]. In this chapter, the neonatal lupus syndrome is summarized and presented.

Epidemiology of Neonatal Lupus Syndrome

AS previously mentioned, SLE can be seen in any age groups including the childhood and neonate. The incidence of connective tissue diseases is much lower in children than adults; however, the clinical picture is more variable. Clinical signs, such as fatigue, fever, or weight loss, may precede any systemic organ involvement and in children, mucocutaneous manifestations develop most frequently during the varying disease course [8]. However, the prevalence of SLE in the young children, especially for infant, is low. However, there is an important syndrome called neonatal lupus syndrome. Cutaneous lupus erythematosus may be related to maternal autoantibody production in the neonatal lupus syndrome, or may occur later in childhood, with or without findings of SLE [9]. Neonatal lupus syndrome is a passively acquired autoimmune syndrome in which pathogenic autoantibodies (anti-SSA/Ro, anti-SSB/La, and both, or rarely anti-U(1)RNP antibodies) are transmitted from a mother to her fetus through the placenta [10-11]. Children born from mothers positive for autoantibodies against SSA/Ro and/or anti-SSB/La ribonucleoproteins may develop heart conduction tissue damage resulting in atrioventricular block and/or transient skin rash, liver enzyme abnormalities and anaemia/thrombocytopenia [10]. Additional transient electrocardiographic abnormalities (sinus bradycardia, QT interval prolongation) have been reported [10]. Such clinical and laboratory manifestations are included in the so-called neonatal lupus syndromes, independently whether the mother is suffering from a systemic autoimmune disease or is totally asymptomatic [10]. The prevalence of the congenital heart block is around 2%, of neonatal rash around 20%, while laboratory abnormalities in asymptomatic babies can be detected in up to 40% of cases [10].

Clinical Presentation of Neonatal Lupus Syndrome

Clinically, SLE is an autoimmune with several organ manifestations. Neonatal lupus, although quite rare, carries a significant mortality and morbidity when the fetal heart is the targeted organ [12]. Anti-SSA/Ro-SSB/La antibodies are present in more than 85% of mothers whose fetuses are identified with congenital heart block in a structurally normal heart, but the risk for a woman who has the candidate antibodies to have a child who has CHB is approximately 2% [12]. Although the precise pathogenic mechanism of injury remains unknown, it is clear that the antibodies alone are insufficient to cause disease and fetal factors are likely contributory [12].

A. Cardiac Manifestation

As previously mentioned, cardiac manifestation is one of the most problematic manifestations of neonatal lupus syndrome. It can lead to death in the worst cases. Pathologically, cardiovascular involvement is common in connective tissue diseases, with relevant implications in terms of morbidity and mortality. Rhythm disturbances, such as conduction defects and tachyarrhythmias, represent a frequent clinical manifestation of connective tissue disease-associated cardiovascular damage and a possible cause of sudden death [13]. Congenital complete heart block can be isolated or can occur in association with other structural heart diseases [14]. Isolated congenital complete heart block is due to transplacental transfer of autoantibodies from mothers with connective tissue disease [14]. Congenital heart block is usually complete, but incomplete blocks, sinus bradycardia and QTc prolongation are also reported [14]. Among connective tissue disease-associated rhythm disorders, congenital heart block, which represents the main feature of neonatal lupus, a rare syndrome related to the transplacental passage of autoantibodies from anti-Ro/SSA-positive mother to their newborns, seems to acknowledge a peculiar mechanism of disease possibly dependent on a direct arrhythmogenicity of anti-Ro/SSA antibodies [13]. Moreover, new anti-Ro/SSA-associated EKG abnormalities have been recently described in children [13]. In 2005, Clancy et al found that reactivity to p200 was a dominant but not uniform anti-Ro 52 response in women whose children had complete heart block [15]. Since exposure to this antibody specificity was observed with a similar frequency in children without CHB born to mothers with anti-Ro 52, additional factors are necessary to convert risk to disease expression [15].

The pathohistologic lesion of autoimmune congenital heart block is fibrosis of the conducting tissue and, in some cases, the surrounding myocardium [16]. The mechanism by which maternal anti-SSA/Ro-SSB/La antibodies initiate and perpetuate inflammation, and eventuate in scarring of the atrioventricular node, is not yet defined [17]. Previous in vitro and in vivo studies suggest that the pathologic cascade is initiated via apoptosis, resulting in translocation of SSA/Ro-SSB/La antigens to the cell surface where they are bound by maternal autoantibodies [16]. Subsequently, the Fc portion of the bound immunoglobulin engages Fcgamma receptors on tissue macrophages, resulting in release of TGF-beta at a threshold favoring a profibrotic milieu and irreversible scarring [16]. This cascade also involves tissue-specific activation of TGF-beta, which promotes the modulation of fibroblasts into myofibroblasts, a scarring phenotype [16-17]. Phagocytosis of opsonized apoptotic cardiocytes is distinct from macrophage pathways engaged in physiologic clearance of dying tissue, which also results in the release of TGFbeta but in the latter case appropriately serves to dampen inflammation [18]. The exaggerated apoptosis (amplified physiologic apoptosis or defective clearance) that is observed in autopsy slides from fetuses who had congenital heart block may provide the pivotal clue to understanding the pathogenicity of the maternal autoantibodies [19]. Dissecting the individual components in this fibrotic pathway should provide insights into the rarity of irreversible injury and should form the basis of rational approaches to prevention and treatment [16-20]. Downregulation of TGFbeta (activation/secretion pathway) may provide the basis of a novel approach to treatment of complete heart block in the future [18].

In addition to rhythmic abnormality, there are also other cardiac manifestations in neonatal lupus syndrome. Acute heart failure is another possible manifestation. This manifestation is usually accompanied with rhythmic abnormality. Endocardititis and myocarditis can be the cause of acute heart failure [21]. The pathogenesis is the same as that of cardiac rhythmic disorder. In these cases, echocardiographically could document heart enlargement, pericardial effusion and moderate insufficiency of either mitral or tricuspid valves [21]. The heart failure can resolve under steroid treatment [21].

B. Cutaneous Manifestation

Cutaneous manifestation is another important manifestation in neonatal lupus syndrome [22]. Unlike the general SLE, the UV light exposure is not a requirement for the development of cutaneous neonatal lupus [23]. Yu et al proposed that that the abnormal expression of both Ro/SSA and La/SSB on the surface membrane of NLE keratinocytes induced the autoantibodies and complements to injure the cells [24]. This complement-mediated cytotoxic effect can be augmented by UV irradiation, a concept not incompatible with the exacerbation of the skin eruption in sun-exposed skin sites [24]. Clinically, periorbital, scalp, and extremity lesions are common in cutaneous neonatal lupus [25]. Crusted lesions usually predominate in male infants [25]. In children selected by cutaneous involvement, thrombocytopenia and hepatic disease are present as frequently as cardiac disease and occurred more frequently in male babies with crusted skin lesions [25]. Weston et al noted that children with cutaneous neonatal lupus should be evaluated for hematologic and hepatic as well as cardiac involvement [25]. According to the work of Nieman et al, the infant's rash often followed UV light exposure; mean age at detection was 6 weeks, and mean duration was 17 weeks [26]. All had facial involvement (periorbital region most common) followed by the scalp, trunk, extremities, neck, and intertriginous areas [26]. The rash resolved without sequelae, 43% of which were untreated [26]. In addition to general skin lesions, telangiectasia is also reported [27]. Neiman et al noted that a quarter of infant's rash had residual sequelae that included telangiectasia and dyspigmentation [26].

C. Hepatic Manifestation

Hepatic manifestation is another important manifestation in neonatal lupus syndrome [22]. Mildly abnormal liver function can be seen [28]. However, some cases can presented severe liver disorders. Three clinical variants of hepatobiliary disease were observed: 1) severe liver failure present during gestation or in the neonatal period, often with the phenotype of neonatal iron storage disease; 2) conjugated hyperbilirubinemia with mild or no elevations of aminotransferases, occurring in the first few weeks of life; and 3) mild elevations of aminotransferases occurring at approximately 2 to 3 months of life [29]. The prognosis for the children in the last 2 categories is excellent [29]. Lee et al noted that clinicians should be aware of the broad range of hepatobiliary disease that may occur in children with neonatal lupus [29]. It should also be noted that hepatobiliary presentation can be exist without other presentations in neonatal lupus [30]. The hepatitis is believed to be due to the passive autoimmune [31-32]. Pathologic changes included giant cell transformation, ductal obstruction, and extramedullary hematopoiesis [33]. Liver involvement has been noted incidentally in children with neonatal lupus erythematosus, but it has generally been attributed to hemodynamic compromise as a result of congenital heart block or systemic toxic reactions [33]. Maternal and infant ANA status should be determined in cases labeled as idiopathic neonatal hepatitis to exclude undiagnosed maternal SLE as a cause of neonatal cholestasis [31].

D. Hematological Manifestation

Hematological manifestation is another important manifestation in neonatal lupus syndrome. Pancytopenia and hemolytic anemia can be seen. Immune thrombocytopenia, disseminated intravascular coagulation (DIC), microangiopathic hemolytic anemia can be seen in the severe cases [34]. This should be differentiate from the product of a preterm twin pregnancy complicated by the development of maternal HELLP (hemolysis, elevated liver enzymes, low platelets) syndrome [35]. The neonatal lupus patient usually has elevated Ro(SSA) and La(SSB) antibody titers, and studies performed on maternal blood usually discloses positive antinuclear antibodies and elevated Ro and La antibody titers [35].

E. Anti-Ro and Anti-La Negative Neonatal Lupus

To our best knowledge, very few cases of neonatal lupus were reported to be negative in anti-Ro and anti-La antibodies. In these cases, the classical signs and symptoms of neonatal lupus can be seen. Other autoantibodies such as RNP and Sm antibodies may play an important role in the pathogenesis of neonatal lupus in these cases [36-37].

DIAGNOSIS OF NEONATAL LUPUS SYNDROME

Similar to general SLE, diagnosis of neonatal lupus syndrome is based on the standard SLE criteria diagnosis. As a rule, the diagnosis of SLE is based on criteria developed by The American Rheumatism Association [38]. This criteria include clinical sign and symptom as well as laboratory results. Transplacental passage of maternal anti-SSA/Ro -SSB/La IgG is thought to be pivotal in inducing tissue damage [39]. Therefore, the anti-Ro and anti-La are the two main markers for diagnosis of neonatal lupus syndrome. The Ro/La system is considered as an heterogeneous antigenic complex, constituted by three different proteins (52 kDa Ro, 60 kDa Ro and La) and four small RNAs particles [40]. Anti-Ro/SSA are the most prevalent specificity among many autoimmune diseases, such as systemic lupus erythematosus (SLE), SS/SLE overlap syndrome, subacute cutaneous LE (SCLE), neonatal lupus and primary biliary cirrhosis [40-41]. In additional to Anti Ro and Anti La, there are also some reports on clinical importance of other autoantibodies. Sheth said that anti-U1RNP antibody might have a correlation to cutaneous lesions of neonatal lupus syndrome [42]. RNP and Sm antibodies are also reported to relate with thrombocytopenia [36-37].

TREATMENT FOR NEONATAL LUPUS SYNDROME

The treatment of neonatal lupus syndrome can apply the general protocol for treatment of SLE in general population. Basically, the immunosuppressive drug is used.

In addition, the treatment for complications should also be considered. However, it should also be noted that some cases of neonatal lupus syndrome can be spontaneous resolved without any therapy.

A. Immunosuppressive Therapy

Usually, immunosuppressive therapy for neonatal lupus is used when the patients have severe manifestations such as severe hepatitis. For severe hepatitis, Lin et al reported that treatment with prednisolone (2 mg/kg/day) for 14 days resulted in dramatic improvement [43]. For cardiac disorder, the prenatal treatment is more preferable.

B. Treatment for Complication of Neonatal Lupus

There are also some specific treatments for complications of neonatal lupus. For conduction defect and heart block, pace maker insertion is required for some neonatal lupus cases with severe conduction defect [44]. For cases presenting with bleeding, replacement therapy is recommended. Blood transfusion to replace blood loss from gastrointestinal bleeding should be done [46]. Additional intravenous immunoglobulin (IVIG) (2 g/kg) combined with corticosteroid (2 mg/kg) is also recommended for those cases [45].

C. Prenatal Immunosuppressant Therapy

Intrauterine steroid treatment in the presence of fetal hydrops and congenital heart block is discussed. The presence of maternal autoantibodies to SS-A/Ro and/or SS-B/La is associated with the development of fetal heart block [46]. There are data suggesting that maternal treatment with steroids might reverse heart block [46-47]. Saleeb et al reported that fluorinated steroids should be considered for fetuses with incomplete block or hydropic changes. Serial echocardiograms are recommended to monitor fetal progress [48]. It remains to be determined whether third-degree block is reversible if therapy is initiated immediately upon detection [48]. Dexamethasone and sympathomimetics may be of some benefit in treating hydrops fetalis [49]. However, in pregnant women with anti-Ro/La antibodies, prophylactic therapy is not indicated but serial echocardiographic analysis is strongly recommended, with emphasis on the mechanical PR interval to identify a reversible block [49].

Prevention for Neonatal Lupus Syndrome

A. Primary Prevention

The best primary prevention is giving the knowledge to all females with SLE. Suggestion for the affected female to avoid pregnancy can be effective tool to cut the cycle to autoantibody transmission to their children

B. Secondary Prevention

Early diagnosis and prompt treatment for neonatal lupus syndrome are two effective secondary prevention. Screening for anti Ro and anti La in the pregnant with SLE can be useful technique to early diagnose possible case of neonatal lupus [50-52]. For those pregnant with positive autoantibodies, closed following up and prompt prenatal treatment when diagnosis of fetal abnormalities should be set. The very early diagnosis of a fetal heart block in bradycardiac fetus by echocardiography is essential for a consecutive therapy with steroids [50]. For anti-SSA/Ro positive pregnant women, echocardiograms should be performed every 2 weeks from 16 to 24 weeks of gestation, and every week in case of past history of complete heart block [51-52]. Electrocardiogram should be performed in the first days of life for all children to detect incomplete complete heart block [51]. By a reduction of the maternal antibodies an improvement of cardial symptoms in the fetus may be achieved in cases with fetal hydrops [50]. Pregnant women at high risk with known connective tissue disease, previous children with congenital heart block, high titers of SS-A-/SS-B-antibodies and immunogenetic predisposition (HLA-DR3) have to be monitored intensively because of the possibility of a prophylaxis with dexamethasone and, in some selected cases, plasmapheresis [50].

References

[1] Fairhurst AM, Wandstrat AE, Wakeland EK. Systemic lupus erythematosus: multiple immunological phenotypes in a complex genetic disease. *Adv Immunol.* 2006;92:1-69.

[2] Kyttaris VC, Krishnan S, Tsokos GC. Systems biology in systemic lupus erythematosus: integrating genes, biology and immune function. *Autoimmunity.* 2006 Dec;39(8):705-9.

[3] Hirose S, Jiang Y, Hamano Y, Nishimura H. Genetic basis of systemic lupus erythematosus. *Drugs Today (Barc).* 2002 Mar;38(3):167-84.

[4] Tsao BP. An update on genetic studies of systemic lupus erythematosus. *Curr Rheumatol Rep.* 2002 Aug;4(4):359-67.

[5] Tsao BP, Grossman JM. Genetics and systemic lupus erythematosus. *Curr Rheumatol Rep.* 2001 Jun;3(3):183-90.

[6] Sallmann DS, Fiebig B, Hedrich CM, Heubner G, Gahr M. Systemic lupus erythematosus in children and adolescents. *Z Rheumatol.* 2006 Nov;65(7):576-586.

[7] Faller G, Thomson PD, Kala UK, Hahn D. Demographics and presenting clinical features of childhood systemic lupus erythematosus. *S Afr Med J.* 2005 Jun;95(6):424-7.

[8] Gensch K, Gudowius S, Niehues T, Kuhn A. Connective tissue diseases in childhood. *Hautarzt.* 2005 Oct;56(10):925-36.

[9] Lee LA, Weston WL. Cutaneous lupus erythematosus during the neonatal and childhood periods. *Lupus.* 1997;6(2):132-8.

[10] Cimaz R, Duquesne A. Neonatal lupus syndromes. *Arch Pediatr.* 2006 May;13(5):473-8.

[11] Iwamoto M. Neonatal lupus syndrome. *Nihon Rinsho Meneki Gakkai Kaishi.* 2005 Feb;28(1):4-9.

[12] Buyon JP, Clancy RM. Neonatal lupus: basic research and clinical perspectives. *Rheum Dis Clin North Am.* 2005 May;31(2):299-313.

[13] Jayaprasad N, Johnson F, Venugopal K. Congenital complete heart block and maternal connective tissue disease. *Int J Cardiol.* 2006 Sep 20;112(2):153-8.

[14] Lazzerini PE, Capecchi PL, Guideri F, Acampa M, Galeazzi M, Laghi Pasini F. Connective tissue diseases and cardiac rhythm disorders: an overview. *Autoimmun Rev.* 2006 May;5(5):306-13

[15] Clancy RM, Buyon JP, Ikeda K, Nozawa K, Argyle DA, Friedman DM, Chan EK. Maternal antibody responses to the 52-kd SSA/RO p200 peptide and the development of fetal conduction defects. *Arthritis Rheum.* 2005 Oct;52(10):3079-86.

[16] Clancy RM, Buyon JP. Autoimmune-associated congenital heart block: dissecting the cascade from immunologic insult to relentless fibrosis. *Anat Rec A Discov Mol Cell Evol Biol.* 2004 Oct;280(2):1027-35.

[17] Buyon JP, Clancy RM. From antibody insult to fibrosis in neonatal lupus - the heart of the matter. *Arthritis Res Ther.* 2003;5(6):266-70.

[18] Buyon JP, Clancy RM. Autoantibody-associated congenital heart block: TGFbeta and the road to scar. *Autoimmun Rev.* 2005 Jan;4(1):1-7.

[19] Clancy RM, Buyon JP. More to death than dying: apoptosis in the pathogenesis of SSA/Ro-SSB/La-associated congenital heart block. *Rheum Dis Clin North Am.* 2004 Aug;30(3):589-602

[20] Clancy RM, Askanase AD, Kapur RP, Chiopelas E, Azar N, Miranda-Carus ME, Buyon JP. Transdifferentiation of cardiac fibroblasts, a fetal factor in anti-SSA/Ro-SSB/La antibody-mediated congenital heart block. *J Immunol.* 2002 Aug 15;169(4):2156-63.

[21] Ferrazzini G, Fasnacht M, Arbenz U, Seger R, Biedermann R, Simma B, Uehlinger J, Dangel P, Fanconi S. Neonatal lupus erythematosus with congenital heart block and severe heart failure due to myocarditis and endocardititis of the mitral valve. *Intensive Care Med.* 1996 May;22(5):464-6.

[22] Bodemer C. Cutaneous manifestations of lupus in children. *Arch Pediatr.* 2004 Jun;11(6):509-11.

[23] Cimaz R, Biggioggero M, Catelli L, Muratori S, Cambiaghi S. Ultraviolet light exposure is not a requirement for the development of cutaneous neonatal lupus. *Lupus.* 2002;11(4):257-60.

[24] Yu HS, Chiang LC, Chang CH, Kang JW, Yu CL. The cytotoxic effect of neonatal lupus erythematosus and maternal sera on keratinocyte cultures is complement-dependent and can be augmented by ultraviolet irradiation. *Br J Dermatol.* 1996 Aug;135(2):297-301.

[25] Weston WL, Morelli JG, Lee LA. The clinical spectrum of anti-Ro-positive cutaneous neonatal lupus erythematosus. *J Am Acad Dermatol.* 1999 May;40(5 Pt 1):675-81.

[26] Neiman AR, Lee LA, Weston WL, Buyon JP. Cutaneous manifestations of neonatal lupus without heart block: characteristics of mothers and children enrolled in a national registry. *J Pediatr.* 2000 Nov;137(5):674-80.

[27] Lin SC, Shyur SD, Wu JY, Huang LH, Yi-Chun. Facial telangiectasia-an unusual complication of neonatal lupus erythematosus: report of one case. *Acta Paediatr Taiwan.* 2004 Jul-Aug;45(4):246-8.

[28] Kanagasegar S, Cimaz R, Kurien BT, Brucato A, Scofield RH. Neonatal lupus manifests as isolated neutropenia and mildly abnormal liver functions. *J Rheumatol.* 2002 Jan;29(1):187-91.

[29] Lee LA, Sokol RJ, Buyon JP. Hepatobiliary disease in neonatal lupus: prevalence and clinical characteristics in cases enrolled in a national registry. *Pediatrics.* 2002 Jan;109(1):E11.

[30] Selander B, Cedergren S, Domanski H. A case of severe neonatal lupus erythematosus without cardiac or cutaneous involvement. Acta Paediatr. 1998 Jan;87(1):105-7.

[31] Evans N, Gaskin K. Liver disease in association with neonatal lupus erythematosus. *J Paediatr Child Health.* 1993 Dec;29(6):478-80.

[32] Lee LA, Reichlin M, Ruyle SZ, Weston WL. Neonatal lupus liver disease. *Lupus.* 1993 Oct;2(5):333-8.

[33] Laxer RM, Roberts EA, Gross KR, Britton JR, Cutz E, Dimmick J, Petty RE, Silverman ED. Liver disease in neonatal lupus erythematosus. *J Pediatr.* 1990 Feb;116(2):238-42.

[34] Hariharan D, Manno CS, Seri I. Neonatal lupus erythematosus with microvascular hemolysis. *J Pediatr Hematol Oncol.* 2000 Jul-Aug;22(4):351-4.

[35] Paton S, Wiss K, Lyon N, Baden L, Gellis SE. Neonatal lupus erythematosus and maternal lupus erythematosus mimicking HELLP syndrome. *Pediatr Dermatol.* 1993 Jun;10(2):177-81.

[36] Horng YC, Chou YH, Tsou Yau KI. Neonatal lupus erythematosus with negative anti-Ro and anti-La antibodies: report of one case. *Zhonghua Min Guo Xiao Er Ke Yi Xue Hui Za Zhi.* 1992 Sep-Oct;33(5):372-5.

[37] Crowley E, Frieden IJ. Neonatal lupus erythematosus: an unusual congenital presentation with cutaneous atrophy, erosions, alopecia, and pancytopenia. *Pediatr Dermatol.* 1998 Jan-Feb;15(1):38-42.

[38] Harvey CJ, Verklan T. Systemic lupus erythematosus: obstetric and neonatal implications. *NAACOGS Clin Issu Perinat Womens Health Nurs*. 1990;1(2):177-85.

[39] Cimaz R, Duquesne A. Neonatal lupus syndromes. *Arch Pediatr*. 2006 May;13(5):473-8.

[40] Franceschini F, Cavazzana I. Anti-Ro/SSA and La/SSB antibodies. *Autoimmunity*. 2005 Feb;38(1):55-63.

[41] Okano T, Satoh M, Akizuki M. Immunologic tests: Anti SS-A/Ro, anti SS-B/La antibody. *Nippon Rinsho*. 2005 Jul;63 Suppl 7:495-8.

[42] Sheth AP, Esterly NB, Ratoosh SL, Smith JP, Hebert AA, Silverman E. U1RNP positive neonatal lupus erythematosus: association with anti-La antibodies? *Br J Dermatol*. 1995 Apr;132(4):520-6.

[43] Lin SC, Shyur SD, Huang LH, Wu JY, Chuo HT, Lee HC. Neonatal lupus erythematosus with cholestatic hepatitis. *J Microbiol Immunol Infect*. 2004 Apr;37(2):131-4.

[44] Ayed K, Gorgi Y, Sfar I, Khrouf M. Congenital heart block associated with maternal anti SSA/SSB antibodies :a report of four cases. *Pathol Biol (Paris)*. 2004 Apr;52(3):138-47.

[45] Chunharas A, Nuntnarumit P, Hongeng S, Chaunsumrit A. Neonatal lupus erythematosus: clinical manifestations and management. *J Med Assoc Thai*. 2002 Nov;85 Suppl 4:S1302-8.

[46] Breur JM, Visser GH, Kruize AA, Stoutenbeek P, Meijboom EJ. Treatment of fetal heart block with maternal steroid therapy: case report and review of the literature. *Ultrasound Obstet Gynecol*. 2004 Sep;24(4):467-72.

[47] Yamada H, Kato EH, Ebina Y, Moriwaki M, Yamamoto R, Furuta I, Fujimoto S. Fetal treatment of congenital heart block ascribed to anti-SSA antibody: case reports with observation of cardiohemodynamics and review of the literature. *Am J Reprod Immunol*. 1999 Oct;42(4):226-32

[48] Saleeb S, Copel J, Friedman D, Buyon JP.Comparison of treatment with fluorinated glucocorticoids to the natural history of autoantibody-associated congenital heart block: retrospective review of the research registry for neonatal lupus. *Arthritis Rheum*. 1999 Nov;42(11):2335-45.

[49] Friedman DM, Rupel A, Glickstein J, Buyon JP. Congenital heart block in neonatal lupus: the pediatric cardiologist's perspective. *Indian J Pediatr*. 2002 Jun;69(6):517-22.

[50] Muller-Ladner U, Benning K, Rother E, Lang B. Neonatal lupus erythematosus as an example of passively acquired autoimmunity. *Immun Infekt*. 1992 Aug;20(4):117-21.

[51] Costedoat-Chalumeau N, Amoura Z, Villain E, Cohen L, Fermont L, Le Thi Huong D, Vauthier D, Georgin-Lavialle S, Wechsler B, Dommergues M, Piette JC. Obstetrical management of patients at risk of neonatal lupus syndrome: review of the literature. *J Gynecol Obstet Biol Reprod (Paris)*. 2006 Apr;35(2):146-56.

[52] Salomonsson S, Dorner T, Theander E, Bremme K, Larsson P, Wahren-Herlenius M. A serologic marker for fetal risk of congenital heart block. *Arthritis Rheum*. 2002 May;46(5):1233-41.

Chapter 13

NEONATAL CELLULAR IMMUNE DEFICIENCY

INTRODUCTION TO IMMUNE DEFICIENCY

Immune system is the basic defense mechanism of human body to the foreign body. Basically, there are two components of immune system: cellular immunity and humoral immunity. Minimally, an immune response is an induced cellular and/or humoral defense mechanism specific for the challenging agent [1]. The system is a cognitive one inasmuch as a second stimulus with the same antigen can specifically induce either an enhanced response (memory) or diminished response (tolerance) [1]. It is almost unbelievable that immune functions as phagocytosis and cytokine production like IL-1 and TNF have already emerged 700 million years ago in starfishes and sponges [2]. Functions--including recruitment of coelomocytes, killing of micro-organisms by lysosome-like enzyme activity, opsonization by complement analogous proteins and oxidative burst function--remained unchanged during phylogenesis and could be found not only in insects but in mammals as well as representatives of innate immunity [2]. Evolution of mechanisms of immune defense has resulted in a variety of strategies [3]. Even unicellular organisms have rich arsenals of mechanisms for protection, such as restriction endonucleases, antimicrobial peptides, and RNA interference.In multicellular organisms, specialized immune cells have evolved, capable of recognition, phagocytosis, and killing of foreign cells as well as removing their own cells changed by damage, senescence, infection, or cancer [3]. Additional humoral factors, such as the complement cascade, have developed that co-operate with cellular immunity in fighting infection and maintaining homeostasis [3]. The cells responsible for the initial antigen-specific recognition in higher vertebrates are clonally restricted T and B lymphocytes [1]. Accessory cells are necessary for the processing and presentation of antigen, and physiologic mediators (cytokines) are essential for proliferation, interaction, and regulation of the system [1].

Basically, the host response involves three different cell types: the phagocytic cell (polymorphs or macrophages), the thymus-dependent (T) lymphocyte, and the thymus-independent (B) lymphocyte-plasma cell line [4]. In human, the humoral immune response plays its role via antibody while the cellular immune response plays its role via lymphocyte. During a humoral immune response, a variety of histological, cellular, and molecular changes occur within the immune system [5]. The immune system makes use of two distinct mechanisms to mount an efficient response against almost every foreign macromolecular substance [6]. First, antibodies with their robust immunoglobulin domain architecture provide a rigid scaffold to support six hypervariable loops, capable of forming highly diverse binding sites [6]. Second, an efficient genetic mechanism has evolved to create sequence diversity at the somatic level in a step-wise process, whereby random recombination of an inherited set of gene segments is followed by hypermutation events [6]. It is proposed that the down regulation of antigen binding receptors in germinal center cells might be designed to exploit anticipated increases in affinity that result from somatic hypermutation in these tissues [5]. This hypothesis is consistent with observed biological changes that occur during an immune response and has bearing on both the mechanism of affinity maturation and generation of immunologic memory [5]. For cellular immune response, the immune process via cytokine from T cell is the hallmark. Basically, T cell development can be divided into many phases. First is an expansion phase prior to TCR rearrangement, which appears to be correlated with programming of at least some response genes for inducibility [7]. Second is a controlled phase of TCR gene rearrangement [7]. Third is the complex process of selection to reach the final step [7]. CD4+ and CD8+ T cell are the two major lymphocyte in cellular immune response. It seems that the auxiliary CD4+ memory cells secrete either IL-2 and interferon gamma (Th1) or IL-4 and IL-5 (Th2) [8]. It has recently been suggested that cytotoxic/suppressor CD8+ cells can also be divided into cells that secrete interferon gamma and no IL-4 (CTL) and cells that secrete IL-4 and IL-5 (suppressor T cells) [8]. CD4+ T cells have their major roles in regulating immune responses, orchestrating both the amplification and deletion of immune cells, particularly CD8+ T cells [9]. These two functions, which represent only an apparent contradiction, appear to be two faces of the same process of regulation [8]. In fact, because the immune response, once activated, needs to be carefully controlled or switched off when the antigenic stimulus is eliminated, the immune system has developed several strategies either to regulate clonal amplification or to avoid useless expansion of activated cells [9].

Immune deficiency is any condition that presents impairment of immune system. Immunodeficiency disorders are a group of disorders in which part of the immune system is missing or defective. Therefore, the body's ability to fight allien foreign bodies is impaired. Our understanding of the immunodeficiency diseases has been facilitated by a number of important advances: (a) The identification of distinct surface determinants on lymphoid cells has led to improved procedures for the isolation of defined lymphoid cell subpopulations; (b) the demonstration that both T- and B-cell populations encompass subpopulations of lymphocytes with different and at times opposing functions; (c) the development of in vitro techniques to assess the functional behavior of isolated lymphoid subpopulations; and (d) the isolation and characterization of genes encoding immunoglobulin molecules and the antigen-specific T-cell receptor, thus defining at a molecular level the mechanisms leading to antibody diversity and to the organization of a recognition unit on T lymphocytes [10]. These advances have not only been important for our understanding of the pathogenesis of immunodeficiency in patients with congenital and acquired immunodeficiency disorders, but have also provided the scientific basis for more rational approaches to the diagnosis and therapy of these disorders [10]. The immunodeficiency can be seen in any age groups.

Neonatal immune deficiency can be seen in medical practice. There are two main types of deficiency: cellular and humoral immune deficiency. In this chapter, the author will focus on the neonatal cellular immune deficiency.

NEONATAL CELLULAR IMMUNE DEFICIENCY

A. Congenital Neonatal Cellular Immune Deficiency

Congenital neonatal cellular immune deficiency can be seen. The immune reactions of man may be subdivided into two main types, the antibody-bound and the cell-bound immunity [11]. The effect of these two systems is realised by two different lymphocyte populations: T- and B-cells, which may show isolated or combined congenital defects and are known as primary immune defects. Antibody deficiency diseases are the by far most frequent congenital diseases [11]. Concerning the frequency the combined and cellular immune defects follow [11]. At present the diagnostic possibilities are already largely developed [11]. Based on thorough knowledge in histophysiologic and dynamic aspects of lymphoid organs, the histopathologic evaluation in cases of suspected immunodeficiency today forms an integral part of the assessment of the immune status [12]. Apart from conventional histologic techniques, advanced technology such as immunohistochemistry and in situ hybridization is applied [12]. This enables analysis of the basic cellular components in various lymphoid tissue compartments, and evaluation of the consequences of the deficiency by the assessment of microorganisms and neoplasia [12].

The summarization on important congenital cellular immune deficiency in neonate will be further presented in this chapter.

1. Thymus Agenesis

Despite advances in modern science, little was known about the thymus, one of the body's key organs in the immune system, until 1961, when Dr. Jacques Miller performed thymectomies in mice [13]. Then it became evident that the thymus played a key role in the body's defense against infection [13]. Since that time, researchers have continued to examine the role of the thymus from fetal life through adulthood [13]. Congenital aplasia of the thymus gland (DiGeorge's syndrome) is an important disorder that lead to the congenital cellular immunodeficiency [14-15]. DiGeorge syndrome is broadly defined as absence or hypoplasia of the thymus due to dysmorphogenesis of the third and fourth pharyngeal pouches in early embryonic life [16]. The DiGeorge syndrome can also affect the heart and parathyroid glands [17]. In complete DiGeorge syndrome, patients have severely reduced T-cell function [17]. However, there are also partial DiGeorge syndrome. Immunological and pathological studies in a case of partial Di George syndrome can reveal an absence of parathyroids, a major hypoplasia of thymus but a relatively moderate decrease in peripheral T-lymphocyte numbers and functions [18]. Deficiency of T lymphocytes has been shown to occur in the presence of as much as 10 to 20% of the normal amount of histologically normal thymic tissue in the partial DiGeorge syndrome [16]. DiGeorge syndrome has now been redefined as a member of a group of disorders that share in common a chromosome deletion resulting in monosomy 22q11 (CATCH-22 or DGA/VCFS) [19]. The basic embryological fault in these disorders is an inadequate development of the facial neural-crest tissues, resulting in defective organogenesis of pharyngeal pouch derivatives that receive cephalic neural-crest contribution to the mesenchmyme [19]. The causes for this maldevelopment are both genetic and extragenetic in origin and the genetic lesions act in concert with random environmental events to produce the ultimate clinical picture [19].

Clinically, affected children show hypoparathyroidism and, because of depressed cell-mediated immunity, serious bacterial, viral and fungal infections [20]. Barrett et al studied the clinical manifestations of 13 cases with DiGeorge syndrome [21]. According to this study [21], ages at the time of presentation ranged from one day to 4 months [21]. Congenital heart defects including truncus arteriosus, ventricular septal defect, interrupted aortic arch, and tetralogy of Fallot commonly brought these infants to medical attention within the first two weeks of life [21]. Abnormal calcium homeostasis was found in all patients [21]. Those patients presenting after the first month of life often had hypocalcemic seizures as the initial clinical manifestation [21]. Immunologic evaluation revealed that total lymphocyte counts, percent T-cells, total T-cells, and T-lymphocyte function ranged from normal to severely depressed [21]. According to another case series by Aglony et al, variable clinical manifestations as well as CD3, CD4 and CD8 T cell counts in patients with DiGeorge syndrome can be found and airway malformations were associated with a higher mortality [22]. For partial DiGeorge syndrome, presentation in the form of repeated infections is rare, since functional cellular immunity is preserved. It usaully presented as a co-incidence in the neonate with congenital heart disease [23].

In some infants with profound immunodeficiency and complete DiGeorge syndrome, the transplantation of thymus tissue can restore normal immune function [17]. Early thymus transplantation - before the development of infectious complications - may promote successful immune reconstitution [17]. Bone marrow transplantation is another alternative practice for treatment of DiGeorge syndrome. Goldsobel et al indicated that minimal thymic influence was necessary for successful bone marrow transplantation and that patients with DiGeorge syndrome with significant T cell deficiency may benefit from this treatment [24]. Borzy et al proposed that bone marrow transplantation could produce peripheral immunoreconstitution without need for significant thymic influence, most likely by providing a source of postthymic T cells, and that bone marrow transplantation should be considered a therapeutic option in patients with DiGeorge syndrome associated with severe T-cell deficiency [25].

2. MHC Class II Deficiency

Major histocompatibility complex (MHC) class II deficiency or CIITA/RFX deficiency or bare lymphocyte syndrome type II is another primary congenital cellular immune deficiency [26]. This syndrome is a hereditary immunodeficiency resulting from the absence of MHCII expression. Considering the central role of MHCII molecules in the development and activation of CD4+ T cells, it is not surprising that the immune system of the patients is severely impaired. This syndrome is the prototype of a "disease of gene regulation.[27]" The genetic lesions responsible for this deficiecny do not lie within the MHC-II locus itself, but reside instead in genes encoding transcription factors controlling MHC-II expression [28].

The affected genes encode RFXANK, RFX5, RFXAP, and CIITA (Class II Transactivator), four regulatory factors that are highly specific and essential for MHCII genes. The first three are subunits of RFX, a trimeric complex that binds to all MHCII promoters [27]. RFXANK, RFX5 and RFXAP are the three subunits of RFX (regulatory factor X), a DNA-binding complex that binds to a conserved cis-acting sequence, the X box, present in the promoters of all MHC-II genes [28]. CIITA is a non-DNA-binding coactivator that functions as the master control factor for MHCII expression [27]. CIITA is a transcriptional coactivator that functions as a master control factor dictating the cell type specificity, induction and level of MHC-II expression [28]. Lentiviral vectors are used for gene therapy in a mouse model of this disease [29]. In addition, by a direct genetic correction approach, a diagnostic test to determine which of the four MHC II genes is defective in new MHC II-deficiency patients has been optimized [29].

The syndrome is characterized by a lack of human leucocyte antigen Class II gene expression, absence of cellular and humoral T-cell immune response to foreign antigens, and impaired antibody productions, resulting in extreme susceptibility to viral, bacterial and fungal infections [30]. In some patients, there is a reduced cell surface expression of human leucocyte antigen Class I molecules also [30]. Clinical onset usually occurrs in the first year of life, usually involving recurrent bronchopulmonary infections and chronic diarrhea [31]. The clinical course is usually complicated by viral meningoencephalitis, hepatitis, cholangitis, and various autoimmune phenomena [31]. According to the study of Klein et al [31], prognosis of this deficiency was very poor: the mean age at the time of death was 4 years and the main cause of death was overwhelming viral infection. Supportive treatment includes intravenous gammaglobulin and prophylaxis against Pneumocystis carinii [30]. The only curative treatment is bone-marrow transplantation [30]. However, Saleem et al found that the patients usually had a generally poor prognosis, with only few alive despite attempts at bone marrow transplantation [32]. Overwhelming viral infection was the predominant cause of death. Alternative transplant strategies or novel therapies are required for these patients [32].

3. TAP-1 or TAP-2 Deficiency (MHC Class I Deficiency)

TAP, the ATP-binding cassette transporter, is a heterodimeric protein composed of TAP-1 and TAP-2. The *TAP1* and *TAP2* genes are closely linked on chromosome 6p21.3 just upstream of the MHC class II locus [33]. MHC class I are cell surface recognition elements expressed on virtually all somatic cells. These molecules sample peptides generated within the cell and signal the cell's physiological state to effector cells of the immune system, both T lymphocytes and natural killer cells [34]. In addition, molecules structurally related to MHC class I, collectively known as MHC-Ib, are more specialized and, in some cases, interact with more limited subsets of lymphoid cells [34]. Because the presentation of peptides by MHC class I molecules is required for normal development and function of cytotoxic CD8 T cells, cases with TAP1 or TAP2 mutations are deficient in these cells [33]. Affected patients often appear healthy in the first years of life [35 - 36],but in late childhood they begin to have recurrent respiratory infections that may lead to bronchiectasis [37]. Currently no satisfactory therapy exists for these patients beyond appropriate treatment of their infections and the attendant respiratory complications [37].

4. Severe Combined Immunodeficiency (SCID)

Severe combined immune deficiencies (SCIDs) are a group of monogenic diseases resulting in profound disturbances of lymphocyte development and function. Affected individuals are prone to life-threatening infections and without treatment do not survive beyond the first year of life [38]. Two major groups of patients have been described, those with or without an associated absence of the enzyme ADA [39]. The heterogeneity of the syndrome is expressed in variable inheritance patterns (particularly defined X-linked or autosomal recessive modes of inheritance), differing clinical presentations, and significant variability in laboratory findings [39]. Some of this heterogeneity of laboratory findings may in fact be contributed to by the high incidence of infection or engraftment of maternal cells in utero [39]. However, profound deficiency of functional attributes of humoral and cell-mediated immunity is more common [39]. Early diagnosis of SCID is critical because chances for successful treatment are highest for infants who have not yet experienced severe opportunistic infections [40]. SCID is a rare disease that can be detected in newborn infants (i.e., those more or equal 1 month of age) by automated blood count and manual differential [40]. Early diagnosis of SCID is rare since, because estimates of the incidence rate range from one in 50,000 to 100,000 births, most pediatricians do not routinely count white blood cells in newborns [40]. Tests for T-cell lymphopenia (TCLP) using dried blood spots (DBS) could be used to identify children with SCID as well as for other immunodeficiencies that would not be apparent until after the child developed an infection [40].

Haematopoietic stem cell transplantation from a well-matched donor offers high rates of survival, but in the absence of a suitable matched donor, parental haploidentical transplants are associated with greater complications, lower success rates and in some instances poor long-term immune recovery [38]. Alternative therapy has been proposed for adenosine deaminase (ADA) deficiency enzyme substitution by polyethylene glycol-ADA [41]. The present novel therapeutic options based on correction of the defective gene by retroviral gene delivery have been used to correct X-linked SCID (SCID-X1) and adenosine deaminase-deficient SCID (ADA-SCID) [38].

B. Acquired Neonatal Cellular Immune Deficiency

Acquired immune deficiency in neonate is more common than congenital immune deficiency. The most common cause of acquired cellular immune deficiency in neonate is the human immunodeficiency virus (HIV) infection. Indeed, HIV infection is one of the most common viral infection in the present day. The worldwide pandemic of human immunodeficiency virus (HIV) casts its shadow on childbirth, especially in developing countries, where the estimated rate of vertical transmission is 15%-40%, compared with 15%-25% in developed countries [42]. Mother-to-child transmission of HIV can occur during pregnancy, in the intrapartum period or postnatally, through breastfeeding [42]. One third of all the breastfed newborn acquire the infection postnatally. The immune-viral dynamics of the transmission of HIV from mother to child are poorly understood. Many recent studies indicate that when wild-type virus is transmitted, an early immune response in the child can lead to the selection of viral escape forms in the first few months of life [43]. These data suggest that adaptive immune surveillance in both mother and child contributes to the pathogenesis of early perinatal HIV [43]. HIV can penetrate through the damaged gastrointestinal mucosa into the newborn blood system [42]. Risk increases during gastrointestinal infections and oral skin lesions [42]. Mother-to-child transmission rate is 3.2 to 100 child years, especially if the mother is infected just before or after labor [42]. The vast majority of HIV-positive children worldwide acquire the infection through vertical transmission [44]. The discovery of successful interventions that interrupt this transmission has been one of the greatest successes in research [44]. The transmission of HIV from an infected mother to her child can be reduced to less than 2 percent by intensive interventions in the antenatal, intranatal and postnatal periods [44]. According to the World Health Organization (WHO), during the year 2003, despite effective antiretroviral (ARV) therapy, there were approximately 700,000 new infections in children worldwide, the majority of whom were from resource-limited countries [45]. Alternative protocols to the long-course and complex regimens of ARV drugs, which in high-income countries have almost eradicated HIV mother to child transmission, have been shown to reduce early transmission rates by 38-50% [45]. However, the accumulation of drug resistance and the long-term toxicities of ARVs mean that alternative approaches need to be developed [45]. Breastfeeding is another important route of HIV transmission from an HIV-infected mother to her infant [45]. However, breastfeeding is an important pillar of child survival and the ideal way of feeding an infant, as well as providing a unique biological and emotional basis for child development [46]. More details on HIV infection in neonate can be seen in any standard HIV textbook.

REFERENCES

[1] Marchalonis JJ, Schluter SF. Development of an immune system. *Ann N Y Acad Sci.* 1994 Apr 15;712:1-12.

[2] Petranyi GG. The complexity of immune and alloimmune response. *Transpl Immunol.* 2002 Aug;10(2-3):91-100.

[3] Danilova N. The evolution of immune mechanisms. *J Exp Zoolog B Mol Dev Evol.* 2006 Nov 15;306(6):496-520.

[4] Collins FM. Cellular antimicrobial immunity. *CRC Crit Rev Microbiol.* 1978;7(1):27-91.

[5] George J, Claflin L. Selection of B cell clones and memory B cells. *Semin Immunol.* 1992 Feb;4(1):11-7.

[6] Skerra A. Imitating the humoral immune response. *Curr Opin Chem Biol.* 2003 Dec;7(6):683-93.

[7] Rothenberg EV. The development of functionally responsive T cells. *Adv Immunol.* 1992;51:85-214.

[8] Pelletier L, Bellon B, Druet P. Cytokines and immune response. *Rev Prat.* 1993 Mar 1;43(5):536-46.

[9] Frasca L, Piazza C, Piccolella E. CD4+ T cells orchestrate both amplification and deletion of CD8+ T cells. *Crit Rev Immunol.* 1998;18(6):569-94.

[10] Waldmann TA. Immunodeficiency: immunoregulation and immunogenetics. *Clin Immunol Immunopathol.* 1986 Jul;40(1):25-36.
[11] Zintl F. Immune defect diseases in childhood. *Z Gesamte Inn Med.* 1977 Oct 15;32(20):523-8.
[12] Huber J, Zegers BJ, Schuurman HJ. Pathology of congenital immunodeficiencies. *Semin Diagn Pathol.* 1992 Feb;9(1):31-62.
[13] Askin DF, Young S. The thymus gland. *Neonatal Netw.* 2001 Dec;20(8):7-13.
[14] Kretschmer R, Say B, Brown D, Rosen FS. Congenital aplasia of the thymus gland (DiGeorge's syndrome). *N Engl J Med.* 1968 Dec 12;279(24):1295-301.
[15] Lischner HW. DiGeorge syndrome(s). *J Pediatr.* 1972 Nov;81(5):1042-4.
[16] Lischner HW, Huff DS. T-cell deficiency in diGeorge syndrome. *Birth Defects Orig Artic Ser.* 1975; 11(1):16-21.
[17] Markert ML, Boeck A, Hale LP, Kloster AL, McLaughlin TM, Batchvarova MN, Douek DC, Koup RA, Kostyu DD, Ward FE, Rice HE, Mahaffey SM, Schiff SE, Buckley RH, Haynes BF. Transplantation of thymus tissue in complete DiGeorge syndrome. *N Engl J Med.* 1999 Oct 14;341(16):1180-9.
[18] Pabst HF, Wright WC, LeRiche J, Stiehm ER. Partial DiGeorge syndrome with substantial cell-mediated immunity. *Am J Dis Child.* 1976 Mar;130(3):316-9.
[19] Hong R. The DiGeorge anomaly. *Clin Rev Allergy Immunol.* 2001 Feb;20(1):43-60.
[20] Hayde M, Braun F, Eibl M, Lachmann D, Chott A, Radaszkiewicz T. DiGeorge syndrome--significance of early diagnosis in cellular immunodeficiency. *Padiatr Padol.* 1985; 20(4):375-80.
[21] Barrett DJ, Ammann AJ, Wara DW, Cowan MJ, Fisher TJ, Stiehm ER. Clinical and immunologic spectrum of the DiGeorge syndrome. *J Clin Lab Immunol.* 1981 Jul;6(1):1-6.
[22] Aglony M, Lizama_M, Mendez C, Navarrete C, Garay F, Repetto G, Perez R, Carrion F, Talesnik E. Clinical findings and immunologic variability in 9 patients with DiGeorge syndrome.: *Rev Med Chil.* 2004 Jan;132(1):26-32.
[23] Martin Mateos MA, Perez Duenas BP, Iriondo M, Krauel J, Gean Molins E. Clinical and immunological spectrum of partial DiGeorge syndrome. *J Investig Allergol Clin Immunol.* 2000 Nov-Dec;10(6):352-60.
[24] Goldsobel AB, Haas A, Stiehm ER. Bone marrow transplantation in DiGeorge syndrome. *J Pediatr.* 1987 Jul;111(1):40-4.
[25] Goldsobel AB, Haas A, Stiehm ER. Bone marrow transplantation in DiGeorge syndrome. *J Pediatr.* 1987 Jul;111(1):40-4.
[26] Morito T. MHC class II deficiency (CIITA/RFX deficiency). *Ryoikibetsu Shokogun Shirizu.* 2000; (32):18-20.
[27] Reith W, Mach B. The bare lymphocyte syndrome and the regulation of MHC expression. *Annu Rev Immunol.* 2001; 19:331-73.
[28] Masternak K, Muhlethaler-Mottet A, Villard J, Peretti M, Reith W. Molecular genetics of the Bare lymphocyte syndrome. *Rev Immunogenet.* 2000; 2(2):267-82
[29] Matheux F, Villard J. Cellular and gene therapy for major histocompatibility complex class II deficiency. *News Physiol Sci.* 2004 Jun;19:154-8.

[30] Elhasid R, Etzioni A. Major histocompatibility complex class II deficiency: a clinical review. *Blood Rev.* 1996 Dec;10(4):242-8.

[31] Klein C, Lisowska-Grospierre B, LeDeist F, Fischer A, Griscelli C. Major histocompatibility complex class II deficiency: clinical manifestations, immunologic features, and outcome. *J Pediatr.* 1993 Dec;123(6):921-8.

[32] Saleem MA, Arkwright PD, Davies EG, Cant AJ, Veys PA. Clinical course of patients with major histocompatibility complex class II deficiency. *Arch Dis Child.* 2000 Oct;83(4):356-9.

[33] Morito T. MHC class I deficiency. *Ryoikibetsu Shokogun Shirizu.* 2000; (32):15-7.

[34] Natarajan K, Li H, Mariuzza RA, Margulies DH. MHC class I molecules, structure and function. *Rev Immunogenet.* 1999; 1(1):32-46.

[35] de la Salle H, Zimmer J, Fricker D, et al: HLA class I deficiencies due to mutations in subunit 1 of the peptide transporter TAP1. *J Clin Investig* 1999; 103:R9.

[36] Moins-Teisserenc HT, Gadola SD, Cella M, et al: Association of a syndrome resembling Wegener's granulomatosis with low surface expression of HLA class-I molecules. *Lancet* 1999; 354:1598.

[37] Primary T Cell Deficiency. Available online at http://www.accessmedicine.com/content.aspx?aID=2147484

[38] Gaspar HB, Thrasher AJ. Gene therapy for severe combined immunodeficiencies. *Expert Opin Biol Ther.* 2005 Sep;5(9):1175-82.

[39] Gelfand EW, Dosch HM. Diagnosis and classification of severe combined immunodeficiency disease. *Birth Defects Orig Artic Ser.* 1983; 19(3):65-72.

[40] Huang H, Manton KG. Newborn screening for severe combined immunodeficiency (SCID): a review. *Front Biosci.* 2005 May 1;10:1024-39.

[41] Fischer A. Severe combined immunodeficiencies. *Immunodefic Rev.* 1992; 3(2):83-100.

[42] Mor Z, Chemtob D, Pessach N, Nitzan-Kaluski D. Human immunodeficiency virus in newborn of infected mothers: pregnancy, breast feeding and prevention. *Harefuah.* 2006 Sep;145(9):682-6, 701.

[43] Pillay T, Phillips RE. Adaptive evolution in perinatal HIV-1. *Best Pract Res Clin Obstet Gynaecol.* 2005 Apr;19(2):211-29.

[44] Merchant RH, Lala MM. Prevention of mother-to-child transmission of HIV--an overview. *Indian J Med Res.* 2005 Apr;121(4):489-501.

[45] Coutsoudis A. Breastfeeding and HIV. *Best Pract Res Clin Obstet Gynaecol.* 2005 Apr;19(2):185-96.

[46] Scarlatti G. Mother-to-child transmission of HIV-1: advances and controversies of the twentieth centuries. *AIDS Rev.* 2004 Apr-Jun;6(2):67-78.

Chapter 14

NEONATAL POLYCYTHEMIA

INTRODUCTION TO POLYCYTHEMIA

A. What is Polycythemia?

Polycythemia is an important hematological disorder. The definition of polycythemia is "a condition characterized by an increased number of erythrocytes in the circulation." This definition is further explained by the laboratory determination of red blood cell parameters, hemoglobin or hematocrit. Generally, women generally have lower hemoglobin values than men. Men have 14.0-18.0 g/dL, while women have levels of 12.0-16.0 g/dL. Basically, examination of the '95% confidence limits' of the 'Nadler' prediction indicates that males with measured red cell mass (RCMs) greater than 25% and females with measured RCMs greater than 30% above their mean normal predicted RCM may be regarded as having polycythaemia [1]. However, the general definition for polycythemia in the general population cannot be applied to the neonate. Neonatal polycythemia is said to be present when the hematocrit greatly exceeds normal values for gestational and postnatal age. This condition affects approximately 1 to 5 percent of newborns [2]. A term infant is considered to be polycythemic if the hematocrit from a peripheral venous sample is greater than 65 percent or the hemoglobin is greater than 22 g/dL [3-6].

Polycythemia can be either primary or secondary. Primary polycythemia generally means primary proliferative polycythemia or polycythemia vera. For diagnosis of primary polycythemia, there are many criteria. One criterion was erythroid colony formation from peripheral blood in a serum-free system, assayed alone and with the addition of recombinant human erythropoietin (Epo), interleukin 3 (IL3), or alpha interferon (alpha-IFN) [7-8]. The remaining criteria are non-culture associated and comprised platelet distribution width (PDW), platelet nucleotide ratio (ATP:ADP), serum erythropoietin and clinical evidence of ischaemic vascular disease [8]. Westwood et al proposed that the combination of culture associated and non-culture associated variables, by use of a simple additive scoring system, gave no false positive and only 6% false negative results in distinguishing primary polycythaemia from other polycythaemias and normal controls in those used in its derivation [8]. For secondary polycythemia, there are several underlying disorders that can cause polycythemia. Secondary polycythemia is defined as an absolute increase in red blood cell mass caused by enhanced stimulation of red blood cell production. Enhanced erythroid stimulation results mainly from hypoxia and kidney disease [9]. Primary polycythemias result from abnormalities expressed in hematopoietic progenitors. In contrast, circulating factors cause secondary polycythemia [10]. There are acquired and congenital causes of both primary and secondary polycythemia [10].

B. Pathophysiology of Polycythemia

The principal function of red bloo cell is the transportation of oxygen. Erythropoiesis proceeds at a rate consistent with the demand for oxygen-carrying capacity, and the major regulator of erythrocyte production is erythropoietin [11]. Erythropoietin, a peptide hormone, is produced primarily by the kidney under control of a tissue oxygenation sensor [11]. Erythrocytosis is a pathologic state characterized by an elevated erythrocyte mass, which may result from increased proliferation of erythroid progenitors due to an intrinsic cellular defect or in response to extrinsic signals [11]. Secondary erythrocytosis results from either physiologically appropriate compensation for inadequate tissue oxygenation or from inappropriate stimulation of erythropoiesis [11]. Erythrocytosis increases oxygen-carrying capacity of the blood, but at high hematocrit levels increased blood viscosity may result in decreased tissue oxygen delivery [11]. Only erythrocytosis produces polycythemia since leukocytes and platelets are present in blood in far smaller proportions [10]. Polycythemia may be due to increased proliferation or decreased apoptosis of erythroid progenitors, or to delayed erythroid differentiation with an increased number of progenitor cell divisions [10]. Prolonged red cell survival, another theoretical cause of polycythemia, has not yet been described and with intact regulatory mechanisms is unlikely to occur [10]. Further research on this topic is recommended.

PRIMARY POLYCYTHEMIA

Polycythemia vera or polycythemia rubra vera is primary polycythemia [12]. Polycythemia vera is a rare, progressive myeloproliferative disorder thought to originate from the clonal expansion of a multipotent haemopoietic stem cell [13]. This disease is characterised by hyperproliferation of the erythroid, myeloid and megakaryocyte lineages in the early phase, anaemia and fibrosis in the spent phase, and with a significant number of patients developing acute myeloid leukaemia in the final phase [13]. Studies investigating the growth factor requirements of committed progenitors have shown hypersensitivity to a number of haemopoietic growth factors (HGF) in vitro and several HGF receptor and signalling molecule alterations have been reported [13]. Overproduction of erythroid cells in polycythemia vera is particular in that it occurs in the absence of a recognizable physiologic stimulus, since circulating serum levels of erythropoietin are normal or lower than normal [14]. Bascially, erythropoietin initiates its cellular response by binding to the erythropoietin receptor (EpoR) expressed on the surface of immature erythroblast [14]. Following ligand binding, EpoR is known to activate a cytoplasmic protein tyrosine kinase, Jak2 which triggers a signal transduction cascade that leads to the development of early erythroid progenitors into mature erythroblast cells [14]. At present, polycythemia rubra vera is classified as one of four diseases collectively called the myeloproliferative disorders of which each disorder leads to an increased production of one or several hematopoietic cell lineages [15]. Progenitors from patients with polycythemia vera display abnormal responses to several growth factors, suggesting the presence of a defect in a signalling pathway common to different growth factors [16]. Although the mechanism underlying the increased erythroid production in polycythemia vera is not well understood, a number of causes have recently came for which may provide insights not only for the pathogenesis of polycythemia vera but also for a fundamental biological process: the mechanism whereby a multipotential stem cell gives rise to a particular cell lineage [14]. The molecular determination of the monoclonal or non-clonal nature of polycythemia cases is now possible in all or almost all cases by study of the methylation pattern of several polymorphic X-linked loci [17]. According to the recent cytogenetic study, the proportion of patients with clonal anomalies, 10-15% at diagnosis, increases with time, myelo-ablative treatments and evolution to myelofibrosis/myeloid metaplasia, so as to be close to 100% in cases with myelodysplasia/acute transformation [17]. A few of the most frequently found non-random anomalies among which in particular trisomy 8 and 9, double trisomy 8+9, 20q- and trisomy of part or totality of 1q had some degree of specificity [17]. Other recurring aberrations, such as 13q- mainly occur in late stages of PV, in which complex, unstable karyotypes were found [17]. Finally none of those anomalies can be considered as a primary lesion [17]. Considering the biomarker, decreased expression of the thrombopoietin receptor c-Mpl, increased expression of the surface receptor polycythemia rubra vera-I, and insulin-like growth factor-I hypersensitivity can be seen in polycythemia vera [18]. These biomarkers, which are not in themselves the causative changes leading to disease development but nonetheless appear intricately linked to the pathological process, may constitute a useful addition to our diagnostic repertoire [19].

Often, people with polycythemia vera have no symptoms for years. Familial cases are very rare and usually manifest in elderly family members. The earliest symptoms usually are weakness, fatigue and headache. Examination usually reveals no abnormality. In some cases, pruritus without any visible skin changes after water exposure can be seen [20]. Most cases presented with the signs and syptoms of the complication of polycythemia vera. The symptoms occurs sporadically with a median age at presentation of 60 years [21-24]. For example, cerebralvascular stroke can be seen [21]. Cerebral infarction is common. Meng et al suggested that stroke secondary to polycythemia vera should be treated with stroke regimen as well as polycythemia vera therapy, and hydroxycarbamide might have stable benefit and few side effects [21]. in addition, they noted that hematocrit assay should be used as a routine item in stroke patients with frequently relapsed [21].Although polycythemia vera is one of the reported causes for cerebral infarction, isolated cerebellar infarction is rarely reported in combination with polycythemia vera [22]. Budd-Chiari syndrome is another frequent described presentation of the cases with polycythemia vera [23]. The Budd-Chiari syndrome, characterized by the obstruction and occlusion of the suprahepatic veins, is a rare typical complication in polycythemia vera patients [24].

The diagnosis of polycythemia vera is commonly based on the WHO criteria [25]. The bone marrow criteria defined by the World Health Organization (WHO) are based on characteristic increase and clustering of morphologically abnormal enlarged megakaryocytes as a pathognomonic clue to describe three distinct phenotypic entities of myeloproliferative disorders (MPDs): (1) essential thrombocythemia (ET), (2) early and overt polycythemia vera (PV) and (3) prefibrotic, early fibrotic, and fibrotic chronic idiopathic myelofibrosis (CIMF-0, 1, 2 and 3) [26]. The acquired V617F mutation in the tyrosine kinase gene JAK2 represents a new molecular marker proving clonality in PV and other chronic myeloproliferative disorders [25]. The new The proposed WHO/European clinical, molecular and pathological (ECMP) criteria reduce the platelet count to the upper limit of normal ($>400x10^9/l$) as inclusion criterion for the diagnosis of thrombocythemia in true ET, early stages of polycythemia vera and prefibrotic CIMF [26]. Phlebotomy is still the treatment of choice to reduce the red cell mass [25]. For polycythemia vera, phlebotomy to control a haematocrit at <0.45 is the cornerstone in treatment [27]. Low-dose acetylsalicylic acid is successful in the primary prophylaxis of vascular complications [25]. Cytoreductive treatment of blood hyperviscosity by phlebotomy or chemotherapy and antiplatelet therapy with low-dose aspirin have dramatically reduced the number of thrombotic complications and substantially improved survival [28]. However, the majority of patients require myelosuppressive therapy during the course of their disease due to progressive myeloproliferation [25]. Hydroxyurea still plays a role in patients of all age groups [25]. Interferon alpha represents an alternative, particularly for younger patients [25]. Currently, there are three agents-hydroxyurea, interferon alfa, and anagrelide-that differ in mechanisms of action and in treating specific phenotypic manifestations of polycythemia vera, suggesting a potential role for combination therapy [29]. As a recommendation, the patients at high risk for thrombohemorrhagic complications all require cytoreduction, as do patients at intermediate risk who are not effectively managed by phlebotomy and low-dose aspirin [29]. In younger patients, the safest and most effective combination treatment appears to be anagrelide plus interferon alfa, while in older patients anagrelide plus hydroxyurea may be effective [29].

NEONATAL POLYCYTHEMIA

A. Molecular Underlying

Actual molecular underlying for neonatal polythemia has not yet been established. However, there are some previous reports on the molecular defect in the neonatal polycythemia. Saggese et al proposed that calcitonin gene-related peptide might be implicated in the circulatory adaptation to extrauterine life [30]. In polycythemic neonates, calcitonin gene-related peptide is probably increased to compensate for blood hyperviscosity; in some cases, high calcitonin gene-related peptide concentrations may induce hypocalcemia, a common complication of polycythemia [30].

B. Pathogenesis

The pathogenesis of neonatal polycythemia is widely discussed. The etiology of polycythemia is related either to intra-uterine hypoxia or secondary to fetal transfusion [31-32]. It is therefore concluded that neonatal polycythemia can result from an excess production of red blood cells (active form) or from an increase in fetal blood volume (passive form) [33]. Intra-uterine hypoxia is a totally unwanted obstetric event. Metabolic acidosis and hypoxia are sequela to asphyxia and can cause profound health effects in postnatal performance because of an abnormal suckling, a reduced absorption of colostrum and inadequate passive transfer of neonatal immunity [34]. Acidosis also cause hypothermia, increased mortality and reduced survival in neonates [34]. One of the first deleterious effects of intrauterine hypoxia is the expulsion of meconium into the amniotic sac leading to meconium staining of the skin, and in severe cases, meconium aspiration into the lungs [34]. Considering the fetal transfusion, polycythemia is an important complication ofm twin twin transfusion syndrome [35-36]. More details can be seen in another chapter in this book. Although it is reasonably common, with an incidence of 1% to 5%, significant symptoms are less frequent and may be more due to predisposing factors such as perinatal asphyxia, intrauterine hypoxia, or hypoglycemia [37]. Infants who are small for gestational age or affected by maternal gestational diabetes are at high risk for the disorder [37]. Fetal macrosomia and infant respiratory distress syndrome, cardiomyopathy, hypoglycemia, hypocalcemia, hypomagnesemia, polycythemia, and hyperviscosity all can occur as a result of maternal hyperglycemia [38]. In addition to general case, a condition similar to the polycythemia vera can also be seen in the neonate [39-40].

C. Clinical Manifestation

Polycythemia is defined as a venous hematocrit above 65% [31]. The relationship between viscosity and hematocrit is almost linear till 65% and exponential thereafter. Increased viscosity of blood is associated with symptoms of hypo-perfusion [31]. Clinical features related to hyperviscosity may affect all organ systems and this entity should be screened for in high-risk infants [31]. Polycythemia maybe symptomatic or asymptomatic [31]. It should be noted that respiratory distress syndrome and cyanonis in newborns (first neonatal week) may be caused by polycythemia [41].

D. Complication

Polycythemia and hyperviscosity are associated with decreases in blood flow to the brain, heart, lung, intestines, and carcass [42]. Renal blood flow is not affected, but renal plasma flow is diminished, resulting in a lower glomerular filtration rate (GFR) [42]. Renal failure can be seen in the worst case. Decreased pulmonary blood flow appears to be the result of hyperviscosity and can result in system hypoxia [42]. This can be corrected by a partial exchange transfusion to lower the hematocrit and viscosity [42]. In addition to the visceral organ, peripheral vascular occlusion can also be the complication of neonatal polycythemia [43]. Gangrenous limb can be seen in the severe cases [43]. Finally, there is also another interesting complication of neonatal polycythemia, hypocalcemia. The underlying genetic of this complication is previously mentioned in this chapter. However, there are many other possible underlying causes. The intense postnatal erythrocyte breakdown will increase the serum level of phosphate [44]. This hyperphosphatemia will decrease calcium ion concentration by their combination and bone deposition, a process allowed by inadequate postnatal parathyroid gland response [44]. The exact pathophysiology for this condition required further research for explanation.

E. Diagnosis and Treatment

Diagnosis of polycythemia in the neonate bases on the previously mentioned hematocrit or hemoglobin level. A term neonate is diagnosed to be polycythemic if the hematocrit from a peripheral venous sample is more than 65 percent or the hemoglobin is more than 22 g/dL [3-6]. Further investigation for the possible underlying cause of neonatal polycythemia must be done in all cases. For treatment, the classical method is phlebotomy [45]. Partial plasma exchange transfusion is the widely used treatment at present [46]. However, concern about the risk of necrotizing enterocolitis following the procedure has recently been raised [46]. Partial exchange transfusion is traditionally used as the method to lower the hematocrit and treat hyperviscosity; however, it is unclear whether this is an effective approach in preventing the long-term neurological consequences [47]. Black et al proposed that there was no significant difference at 1 year between the polycythemic infants who had received partial plasma exchange transfusion and those given only symptomatic care [48]. At 2 years, the group receiving partial plasma exchange transfusion had fewer neurologic diagnoses and fine motor abnormalities [48]. The new technique as dilutional partial exchange transfusion with 5% albumin is also proposed. Safety and lack of complications make human albumin solution is superior to human plasma for exchange transfusion in neonatal polycythemia [49]. According to the recent metanalysis, crystalloid solutions are as effective as colloid solutions for partial exchange transfusion [50]. When crystalloid solutions are used for this purpose, there is no risk of transmission of blood-borne diseases, there is no risk of anaphylaxis, they are rapidly and easily available, and are less expensive [50]. The use of crystalloid should become the standard for partial exchange transfusion [50].

Hyperviscosity Syndrome in the Neonate

Hyperviscosity syndrome is an important condition in hemato-oncology. It is sometimes called as "thick blood syndrome." Polycythemia must be distinguished from hyperviscosity, which is defined as a blood viscosity greater than 12 centipoise, measured at a shear rate of 11.5 per sec or greater than 6 centipoise, measured at a shear rate of 106 per sec [2,51]. However, blood viscosity determination is not feasible for general medical laboratory. Therefore, the indirect determination by hematocrit value is used. Common clinical manifestations of the hyperviscosity syndrome are bleeding from mucosal membrane, retinopathy, visual disturbance and neurological disorders [52]. These changes can be lethal, and early recognition is important for the proper therapy [52]. This condition is frequently detected in the patients with multiple myeloma. Five to 10 percent of patients with multiple myeloma are suffered from the hyperviscosity syndrome because of increased serum viscosity due to the presence of myeloma protein [52]. In general adult, hyperviscosity syndrome is usually an oncological complication. This can lead to several complications in cancerous patients. However, in neonate, it is usually a complication of neonatal polycythemia [53]. Of the hyperviscous babies 41% had plethoric lungs, 12% abnormal electrocardiograms, 9% were hypocalcaemic and 30% hypomagnesaemic [54]. In most of the infant patients with hyperviscosity syndrome, there was no demonstrable abnormal proteolysis in the circulation., however, in such infants the normally low levels of antithrombin III (heparin cofactor activity) in combination with the impairment of the microcirculation might increase the risk of thrombotic complications [55]. Simple screening of all neonates four hours after birth is recommended so that treatment can be given early [56]. The treatment for this condition is previously described in the treatment of neonatal polycythemia. Blood letting is the classical method that is out of date. Hemodilution, preferably with plasma, is therefore advocated in the symptomatic patients [55].

REFERENCES

[1] Pearson TC, Glass UH, Wetherley-Mein G. Interpretation of measured red cell mass in the diagnosis of polycythaemia. *Scand J Haematol.* 1978 Aug;21(2):153-62.

[2] Garcia-Prats JA. Neonatal polycythemia. Available online at http://patients.uptodate.com/topic.asp?file=pedi_hem/9995

[3] Oski, FA, Naiman, JL. Polycythemia and hyperviscosity in the neonatal period. In: *Hematologic Problems in the Newborn*, 3rd ed, Oski, FA (Ed), WB Saunders, New York 1982. p.87.

[4] Wiswell TE, Cornish JD; Northam RS. Neonatal polycythemia: frequency of clinical manifestations and other associated findings. *Pediatrics* 1986 Jul;78(1):26-30.

[5] Stevens, K, Wirth, FH. Incidence of neonatal hyperviscosity at sea level. *J Pediatr* 1980; 97:118.

[6] Ramamurthy, RS. Neonatal polycythemia and hyperviscosity; state of the art. *Perinatology-Neonatology* 1979; 3:38.

[7] Dudley JM, Westwood N, Leonard S, Eridani S, Pearson TC. Primary polycythaemia: positive diagnosis using the differential response of primitive and mature erythroid progenitors to erythropoietin, interleukin 3 and alpha-interferon. *Br J Haematol.* 1990 Jun;75(2):188-94.

[8] Westwood N, Dudley JM, Sawyer B, Messinezy M, Pearson TC. Primary polycythaemia: diagnosis by non-conventional positive criteria. *Eur J Haematol.* 1993 Oct;51(4):228-32.

[9] Balcerzak SP, Bromberg PA: Secondary polycythemia. *Semin Hematol* 1975 Oct; 12(4): 353-82.

[10] Prchal JT. Molecular biology of polycythemias. *Intern Med.* 2001 Aug;40(8):681-7.
[11] Golde DW, Hocking WG, Koeffler HP, Adamson JW. Polycythemia: mechanisms and management. *Ann Intern Med.* 1981 Jul;95(1):71-87.
[12] Bilgrami S, Greenberg BR. Polycythemia rubra vera. *Semin Oncol.* 1995 Aug;22
[13] Butcher C, D'Andrea RJ. Molecular aspects of polycythemia vera (review). *Int J Mol Med.* 2000 Sep;6(3):243-52.
[14] Fernandez-Luna JL, Silva M, Richard C, Sanz C, Benito A. Pathogenesis of polycythemia vera. *Haematologica.* 1998 Feb;83(2):150-8.
[15] Pahl HL. Towards a molecular understanding of polycythemia rubra vera. *Eur J Biochem.* 2000 Jun;267(12):3395-401.
[16] Tanzer J. Pathogenesis of polycythaemia vera. *Blood Rev.* 1997 Dec;11(4):224-32.
[17] Tanzer J. Clonality and karyotype studies in polycythemia vera. *Nouv Rev Fr Hematol.* 1994 Apr;36(2):167-72.
[18] Pahl HL. PRV-1 mRNA expression and other molecular markers in polycythemia rubra vera. *Curr Hematol Rep.* 2003 May;2(3):231-6.
[19] Pahl HL. Diagnostic approaches to polycythemia vera in 2004. *Expert Rev Mol Diagn.* 2004 Jul;4(4):495-502.
[20] Abdel-Naser MB, Gollnick H, Orfanos CE. Aquagenic pruritus as a presenting symptom of polycythemia vera. *Dermatology.* 1993;187(2):130-3.
[21] Meng R, Zhou J, Ji XM, Li LM, Jia JP, Yang BF. The diagnosis and treatment of polycythemia rubra vera manifesting as acute cerebral stroke. *Zhonghua Nei Ke Za Zhi.* 2006 May;45(5):366-8.
[22] Abdel-Naser MB, Gollnick H, Orfanos CE. Aquagenic pruritus as a presenting symptom of polycythemia vera. *Dermatology.* 1993;187(2):130-3.
[23] Cario H, Pahl HL, Schwarz K, Galm C, Hoffmann M, Burdelski M, Kohne E, Debatin KM. Familial polycythemia vera with Budd-Chiari syndrome in childhood. *Br J Haematol.* 2003 Oct;123(2):346-52.
[24] Slakey DP, Klein AS, Venbrux AC, Cameron JL. Budd-Chiari syndrome: current management options. *Ann Surg.* 2001 Apr;233(4):522-7.
[25] Lengfelder E, Merx K, Hehlmann R. Diagnosis and therapy of polycythemia vera. *Semin Thromb Hemost.* 2006 Apr;32(3):267-75
[26] Michiels JJ, De Raeve H, Hebeda K, Lam KH, Berneman Z, Schroyens W, Schwarz J. WHO bone marrow features and European clinical, molecular, and pathological (ECMP) criteria for the diagnosis of myeloproliferative disorders. *Leuk Res.* 2007 Mar 14;
[27] Penninga EI, Bjerrum OW. Polycythaemia vera and essential thrombocythaemia: current treatment strategies. *Drugs.* 2006;66(17):2173-87.
[28] Barbui T, Finazzi G. Evidence-based management of polycythemia vera. *Best Pract Res Clin Haematol.* 2006;19(3):483-93.
[29] Gilbert HS. Modern treatment strategies in polycythemia vera. *Semin Hematol.* 2003 Jan;40(1 Suppl 1):26-9.
[30] Saggese G, Bertelloni S, Baroncelli GI, Cipolloni C. Elevated calcitonin gene-related peptide in polycythemic newborn infants. *Acta Paediatr.* 1992 Dec;81(12):966-8.

[31] Upadhyay A, Aggarwal R, Deorari AK, Paul VK. Polycythemia in the newborn. *Indian J Pediatr*. 2002 Jan;69(1):79-82.

[32] Danish FH. Neonatal polycythemia. *Prog Hematol*. 1986;14:55-98.

[33] Armentrout DC, Huseby V. Polycythemia in the newborn. *MCN Am J Matern Child Nurs*. 2003 Jul-Aug;28(4):234-9

[34] Alonso-Spilsbury M, Mota-Rojas D, Villanueva-Garcia D, Martinez-Burnes J, Orozco H, Ramirez-Necoechea R, Mayagoitia AL, Trujillo ME. Perinatal asphyxia pathophysiology in pig and human: a review. *Anim Reprod Sci*. 2005 Nov;90(1-2):1-30.

[35] Seng YC, Rajadurai VS. Twin-twin transfusion syndrome: a five year review. *Arch Dis Child Fetal Neonatal Ed*. 2000 Nov;83(3):F168-70.

[36] Ongkie AS. Syndrome of hyperviscosity in the neonate (literature review). *Paediatr Indones*. 1974 Nov-Dec;14(11-12):232-48.

[37] Werner EJ. Neonatal polycythemia and hyperviscosity. *Clin Perinatol*. 1995 Sep;22(3):693-710.

[38] Jones CW. Gestational diabetes and its impact on the neonate. *Neonatal Netw*. 2001 Sep;20(6):17-23.

[39] Athanasiou-Metaxa M, Economou M, Tsantali C, Koussi A, Gombakis N. Congenital erythrocytosis with increased erythropoietin level. *J Pediatr Hematol Oncol*. 2002 Mar-Apr;24(3):234-6.

[40] Poggi V, Migliorati R, Fiore M, Amoroso R, Ghio R, Fiorillo A. Polycythemia vera: a new case report with onset in infancy. *Haematologica*. 1984 Jul-Aug;69(4):458-63.

[41] Frisch H, Schabel F. Polycythemia in the newborn infant (author's transl). *Padiatr Padol*. 1977;12(3):294-300.

[42] Rosenkrantz TS. Polycythemia and hyperviscosity in the newborn. *Semin Thromb Hemost*. 2003 Oct;29(5):515-27.

[43] Letts M, Blastorah B, al-Azzam S. Neonatal gangrene of the extremities. *J Pediatr Orthop*. 1997 May-Jun;17(3):397-401.

[44] Merlob P, Amir J. Pathogenesis of hypocalcemia in neonatal polycythemia. *Med Hypotheses*. 1989 Sep;30(1):49-50.

[45] Kontras SB. Polycythemia and hyperviscosity syndromes in infants and children. *Pediatr Clin North Am*. 1972 Nov;19(4):919-33.

[46] Rothenberg T. Partial plasma exchange transfusion in polycythaemic neonates. *Arch Dis Child*. 2002 Jan;86(1):60-2

[47] Schimmel MS, Bromiker R, Soll RF. Neonatal polycythemia: is partial exchange transfusion justified? *Clin Perinatol*. 2004 Sep;31(3):545-53, ix-x.

[48] Black VD, Lubchenco LO, Koops BL, Poland RL, Powell DP. Neonatal hyperviscosity: randomized study of effect of partial plasma exchange transfusion on long-term outcome. *Pediatrics*. 1985 Jun;75(6):1048-53.

[49] Levy I, Merlob P, Ashkenazi S, Reisner SH. Neonatal polycythaemia: effect of partial dilutional exchange transfusion with human albumin on whole blood viscosity. *Eur J Pediatr*. 1990 Feb;149(5):354-5.

[50] Dempsey EM, Barrington K. Crystalloid or colloid for partial exchange transfusion in neonatal polycythemia: a systematic review and meta-analysis. *Acta Paediatr.* 2005 Nov;94(11):1650-5.

[51] Swetnam SM, Yabek SM; Alverson DC. Hemodynamic consequences of neonatal polycythemia. *J Pediatr* 1987 Mar;110(3):443-7.

[52] Hashimoto T. Hyperviscosity syndrome. *Nippon Rinsho.* 1995 Mar;53(3):695-8.

[53] Black VD. Neonatal hyperviscosity syndromes. *Curr Probl Pediatr.* 1987 Feb;17(2):73-130.

[54] Malan AF, de V Heese H. The management of polycythaemia in the newborn infant. *Early Hum Dev.* 1980 Dec;4(4):393-403.

[55] Henriksson P. Hyperviscosity of the blood and haemostasis in the newborn infant. *Acta Paediatr Scand.* 1979 Sep;68(5):701-4.

[56] Wesenberg RL. Neonatal 'thick blood' syndrome. *Hosp Pract.* 1978 May;13(5):137-40, 145.

Chapter 15

NEONATAL BLOOD INFECTION

INTRODUCTION

The word "blood infection" means a common group of hematologic and infectious disorders. Good examples of blood infections are malaria and babesiosis. Most blood infections are endemic in tropical countries and become important public health threaten for the developing countries. However, the blood infections can be seen in non tropical countries as well. There is still limited knowledge on this topic while the wider distribution of the disorder due to the globalization can be expected. Most practitioners should realize and urge to get the information on this topic. Similar to other types of infection, the blood infection has two important basic compartments: pathogen and host. Early views of pathogenicity and virulence were primarily pathogen centered and were based on the assumption that these characteristics were intrinsic properties of microorganisms, although it was recognized that pathogenicity was neither invariant nor absolute [1]. For host, the host defense mechanism is a basic response to the foreign invader. This defense mechanism can result in having or having not infection. However, new information about the attributes of microbes and their hosts resulted in the understanding that the host-pathogen interaction does not always result in disease [2].

Vertical transmission is the transfer of a pathogen from a parent, usually the mother, to the offspring through reproduction. Basically, the transplacental transmission can be occurred if there is an infection within the mother. Usually, the mothers get infection during the pregnancy, especially in the third trimester adjunctive to the labor period. Infection in early infection rarely results in transplacental transmission and congenital infection since the affected fetus usually dies in utero and abortion is the result. An important considerable fact for the tranplacental transmission is that the pathogen has to pass across the placenta from mother to the fetus. The main determinants for this event are size of pathogen and placenta sieve pore size. The pathogen must have smaller size than the pore size [3]. However, some additional mechanism such as transformation of parasite shape and direct invasion into the tissue of placenta and cross to the fetus can also be seen. The vertical transmission is the important mode of transmission bringing to the neonatal blood infection. However, other modes of transmission should also not be overlooked. In this chapter, the neonatal blood infection is summarized and presented.

NEONATAL MALARIA

Malaria is a mosquito-borne parasitic infection. It can be said that malaria is a very important tropical mosquito-borne infectious disease. Malaria is caused by protozoan parasites of the genus Plasmodium. Four species of *Plasmodium, Plasmodium falciparum, Plasmodium vivax, Plasmodium ovale* and *Plasmodium malariae* can produce the human disease in its various forms. Although there have been many efforts for decades to produce a vaccine to combat this infection, few have been able to meet the challenges posed by the unusual interplay between this virus and its human host. According to the globalization at present, the malaria becomes an emerging infectious problem not only to the tropical but also to the non-tropical countries. Malarial infections are one of the most important mosquito-borne diseases in the world. With an annual incidence of 300-500 million clinically manifest cases and a death toll of 1.1-2.7 million, malaria is still one of the most important communicable diseases [4].

Some pregnant women may also be susceptible to dengue and if they experience malaria, the vertical transmission of the plasmodium protozoa to their babies can be expected. The intrapartum malaria is an interesting tropical intrapartum infection. There are some previous reports on this infection. In areas of stable endemicity, the main consequences are maternal anemia and intra-uterine growth retardation resulting in low birthweight (LBW) particularly after first pregnancy [5]. In addition, recent studies have demonstrated that frequency and severity of placental malaria are greater in pregnant women with concurrent HIV infection [5]. The intrapartum malaria can bring several intrapartum complications, of which cerebral malaria is the most serious form [5-6]. Okoko et al proposed that the significantly higher risk of maternal malaria and consequences in primigravidae compared with multigravidae suggested that there were more to mere immunosuppression in pregnancy [50]. They noted that malaria infection of placenta caused a shift from Th2 to Th1 cytokine profile that might be detrimental to pregnancy [6]. They also proposed that increased susceptibility in the first pregnancy could be explained by the absence of anti-adhesion antibody in the primigravida that was being exposed for the first time to a different strain of malaria parasite sub-population that adhere exclusively to chondroitin sulfate A and hyaluronic acid (HA) in the placenta [6]. Vertical transmission due to intrapartum malaria was mentioned.

In congenital anemia, affected children are usually presented with severe anemia and hepatosplenomegaly [7]. Marques *et al* said that despite congenital malaria was being considered a rare event it was a preventable disease and these cases should draw attention to the importance of adequate treatment during pregnancy [7]. In 2006, Wiwanitkit performed a literature review of the reports of congenital malaria in Thailand in order to summarize the characteristics of this infection among Thai patients [8]. According to this study, there have been at least six reports in the literature of 27 cases of congenital malaria infection in the Thai population, of which no case was lethal. There were 22 vivax (81.5%) and five falciparum (18.5%) malarial cases [8]. According to this study, it can be seen that congenital malaria may occur in the absence of clinical symptoms in mothers as well as their children [8]. Concerning the species of malaria, the vivax malaria is more common in this case series [8]. This study implies the importance of congenital malaria in endemic area. Ahmed *et al* noted that the diagnosis of congenital malaria should be considered in infants with suspected congenital infection who were born to mothers with a history of living in or travel to endemic areas [9].

NEONATAL BABESEOSIS

Human babesiosis is caused predominantly by *Babesia microti* and *Babesia divergens*, a protozooan parasites of red blood cells [10]. Both are transmitted by *Ixodes ricinus* ticks, also the primary vector of Lyme disease [10]. Babesia is a tick-transmitted protozoal parasite that can cause malaria-like symptoms and hemolytic anemia [11]. Clinical manifestation varied widely from asymptomatic infection to a serve rapidly fatal disease [10]. Asplenic, elderly, and immunocompromised patients are at greatest risk for severe disease; however babesiosis can be serious in immunologically normal persons [11]. The main clinical manifestations of human bebesiosis are due to the rupture of infected red blood cells as previously mentioned. According to this situation, the hemoglobinemia, hemoglobinuria, hemolytic jaundice and renal failure can be seen in the infected patients. Concerning the lysis of red blood cells, the increasing number of babesia within the cell is the main cause and lysis of red blood cells is for entering new uninfected red blood cells. Similar to other infection, when an organism enters into human bodies, host defense will occur. Immunological reaction to babesia can be seen. *Babesia bovis* and its bovine host interact in many ways, resulting in a range of disease and infection phenotypes [12]. There are some cases of congenital babeseosis [13-14]. But it is not common. However, as previously stated, there are also other mode of transmissions for neonatal babeseosis including blood transfusion (most common) and vector transmission [14]

NEONATAL LEISHMANIASIS

Leishmaniasis is an important tropical vector-borne disease. There are two common forms of leishmaniasis, cutaneous and visceral forms. Leishmanioses are a group of parasitic diseases that affect man and other mammals. They are caused by different species of trypanosomatids of the genus Leishmania [15-16]. Leishmaniasis represents a complex of diseases with a clinical and epidemiological diversity [17]. Leishmaniasis remains a severe public health problem and its burden is increasing [3]. The disease is caused by a parasite belonging to the genus Leishmania [17]. Approximately 350 billion people in 88 different countries are thought to be infected with Leishmania spp [17]. The distribution of this re-emerging disease, which is found throughout the world (except in Antarctica), is influenced by various factors linked to both human activity and climatic change [16]. The heteroecious life cycle of the Leishmania includes an invertebrate host (sandflies of the Phlebotomidae family) [16-18]. The dog is the main reservoir for this disease. The pathogenesis is governed by parasite and host factors and immunoinflammatory responses, the clinical spectrum of leishmaniasis encompasses subclinical (inapparent), localised (skin lesions), and disseminated infection (cutaneous, mucosal, or visceral) [19]. Symptomatic disease is subacute or chronic and diverse in presentation and outcome [19].

Of interest, vertical transmission of leishmaniasis is also reported [20]. Infection with *Leishmania chagasi* during pregnancy is rare and deserves special attention since little information is available regarding the occurrence of visceral leishmaniasis during gestational period and the real possibility of vertical transmission of this disease [21]. Vertical transmission of leishmaniasis is possible and the institution of treatment is imperative in cases of pregnant women with kala-azar. Amphotericin B is strongly recommended as the first choice drug due to its fewer maternal-fetal adverse effects [21]. Visceral leishmaniasis has to be considered in children with fever, pancytopenia, and splenomegaly, even if the child has not been to an endemic area and even if there is no evidence of the disease in his environment, because leishmaniasis can be transmitted congenitally from an asymptomatic mother to her child [20]. It is important to follow-up of infants born to mothers with leishmaniasis [22]. However, as previously stated, there are also other mode of transmissions for neonatal babeseosis including blood transfusion (most common) and vector transmission [23].

Neonatal Trypanosomiasis

Trypanosomiasis is an important vector borne blood infection. The pathogenic organisms causing trypanosomiasis is the parasite in the genus Trypanosoma. In the peripheral blood smear, it is usually characterized by an undulating membrane. There are three main medically important species: *Trypanosoam brucei gambiense*, *T. brucei rhodesiense* and *T. cruzi*. There are three main types of trypanosomiasis: African sleeping sickness caused by *Trypanosoam gambiense*, East African sleeping sickness caused by *T. rhodesiense* and Chagas disease caused by *T. cruzi*. For the vertical transmission of trypanosomiasis, there are some reports on this topic. Velarde performed a preliminary study performed on 3000 pregnant of Arequipa shows serological positives in 22 (0.7%) and only a newborn positive at IgM [24]. This result indicates a probable low rate of congenital transmission and necessary to perform more studies [24]. Mendoza Ticona reported a similar low possibility of vertical transmission in Peru [25]. Luquetti also reported the same situation in Brazil [26]. However, there are some reports on the opposite findings. Sanchez Negrette et al performed a work to study the presence of *T. cruzi* infection in children who were born to infected mothers and in the children's siblings to evaluate the epidemiologic risk factors associated with congenital transmission of Chagas' disease [27]. According to this work, siblings of an infant infected with *T. cruzi* are at high risk for infection themselves and, even in the absence of symptoms, should also be screened for infection [27]. The findings of family clustering of infection and of second-generation congenital infection in vector-free areas suggest that new modalities of transmission, other than classic vector-borne spread, may occur both in endemic and in nonendemic areas [27]. Preventing vertical transmission of *T.cruzi* is not possible, but it can be precociously detected, permitting mother and child to be incorporated into the medical attention system, and so allowing the newborns treatment with practically 100% efficacy

[28]. Exacerbation of infection during pregnancy is also considered as a possible risk factor for transmission [30]. Besides, a relationship between the frequency of transmission and gestational age is presented [30]. Concerning breast-feeding, the risk of transmission is directly related to the acute phase of maternal disease and bleeding nipples [30]. The implementation of an early strategy of detection for an effective and opportune treatment acquires great relevance as a Public Health measure [28-29]. Trypanosoma cruzi-specific IgG is recommended as a screening for the endemic area [31].

NEONATAL TOXOPLASMOSIS

Toxoplasmosis is a parasitic infestation mainly caused by *Toxoplasma* spp. parasite of animals [32-33]. It is classified as an obligate intracellular parasite [32]. The main pathogenic protozoan was first observed in the North African rodent (*Ctenodactylus gundi*) by Nicolle and Manceaux in 1908 therefore it was later given the name "*Toxoplasma gondii*". Since the first discovery, there have been continuously reported on detection of disease in other animals including rabbit, squirrel, dog, monkey and pigeon. *T. gondii* has been found worldwide in many species, including carnivorous and herbivorous mammals and birds. It has also been found in every population group of humans investigated [34]. However, the definitive host was shown to be cats, which have been associated with transmission of the parasite in every population investigated [34]. At present, this disease can be seen all over the world. In addition, it becomes an emerging for humans in the era of human immunodeficiency virus (HIV) infection.

Congenital toxoplasmosis is an important congenital infection. Toxoplasma is an important member of the well-known TORCH agents. Pregnant women who acquire infection from *T. gondii* usually remain asymptomatic, although they can still transmit the infection to their fetuses with severe consequences [35]. Given the asymptomatic nature of most Toxoplasma infections, primary prevention in pregnant women may lower the risk of congenital toxoplasmosis [35]. Both consumption of undercooked meat and unprotected contact with soil are independent risk factors for *T. gondii* seroconversion during pregnancy, while contact with cat litter may pose a risk in certain situations [35]. Serologic tests are used to diagnose acute *T. gondii* infection in pregnant women [36]. Because false-positive tests occur frequently, serologic diagnosis must be confirmed at a Toxoplasma reference laboratory before treatment with potentially toxic drugs is considered [36]. In many instances, congenital toxoplasmosis can be prevented by educating pregnant women and other women of childbearing age about not ingesting raw or undercooked meat, using measures to avoid cross-contamination of other foods with raw or undercooked meat, and protecting themselves against exposure to cat litter or contaminated soil [36]. Congenital toxoplasmosis remains important causes of deafness, vision loss, and behavioral or neurologic disorders among children worldwide [37]. Chorioretinitis, hydrocephalus, intracranial calcifications, and convulsions are the typical presentation of classic congenital toxoplasmosis. Serology is the most common method of diagnosing neonatal infection, but more complex tests are also utilized. The prognosis for the untreated infant is poor; however, when antibiotic therapy is started early, the rate of sequelae is reduced significantly [38]. In general, prenatal therapy of congenital toxoplasmosis is beneficial in reducing the frequency of infant infection. Therapies are based primarily on spiramycin because of the relative lack of toxicity and high concentrations achieved in the placenta [39]. Clindamycin is the standard drug for chemoprophylaxis in newborn infants, and is directed at preventing the occurrence of retinochoroiditis as a late sequel to congenital infection [39].

Congenital toxoplasmosis becomes an important public health threat for many countries in the present AIDS era. Many newborn children in developing countries have congenital anomalies attributable to *T. gondii* [40]. The toxoplasma is included in the TORCH agent, which can be transmitted via placenta. The screening for this infection is recommended. As a consensus, the European experience does not permit conclusions either in favor of or against a programme for the systematic screening of congenital toxoplasmosis [41]. However, cost-benefit analysis plays a very important role in determining whether such a programme should be implemented. Parameters such as the security of diagnosis (standardization of methods, quality and experience of the laboratories) and the monitoring of cases (definition, multidisciplinary approach to the surveillance and long-term treatment of patients, national collection of case reports, evaluation of the program) are indispensable for the implementation of an effective surveillance system [41]. However, neonatal screening for congenital toxoplasmosis by IgM anti-Toxoplasma determination in dried blood from the heel is practiced in many countries [42-44]. Carvalheiro et al reported their experience in the screening in Brazil [45]. They found that the disease incidence was estimated to be 3.3/10,000, indicating the need for preventive measures [45]. They concluded that neonatal screening was feasible, but screening tests with a better performance were required; positive screening results had to be carefully confirmed [45]. In addition to the heel sampling for screening, there is a new attempt to apply the cord blood sampling [46-47]. Cord blood screening is a helpful tool for the detection of infants probably infected with Toxoplasma gondii, if serological data of the mothers are not available [47]. Signorell et al proposed that because toxoplasma specific IgA/IgM antibodies in cord blood identified almost all infected children, screening at birth might be more cost effective than during pregnancy [46].

Neonatal Filariasis and Dirofilariasis

Filariasis and dirofilariasis are important tropical mosquito-borne parasitic infections. Filariasis is the name of name for a group of tropical diseases caused by various thread-like parasitic roundworms and their larvae. Filariasis presents with fever, chills, headache, and skin lesions in the early stages and, if untreated, it can progress to include gross enlargement of the limbs and genitalia in a condition called elephantiasis. Several different types of worms are mentioned as causes of filariasis but the common species include the following: *Wucheria bancrofti, Brugia malayi, Onchocerca volvulus, Loa loa, Mansonella streptocerca, Dracunculus medinensis*, *Mansonella pustans*, and *Mansonella ozzardi*. However, it should be noted that not all human filariasis diseases are mosquito-borne. Concerning dirofilariasis, it is described as infection with roundworms of the genus dirofilaria, usually in animals, especially dogs, but occasionally in man [48]. Cats and dogs are the main hosts suffering from dirofilariasis. Since the filarial parasite is a large microorganism, therefore, transmission via placenta seems impossible. However, there are some case reports on vertical transmission of filariasis [49-51]. In 1995, Fonticiella et al presented the case of a newborn with intracranial extra-axial collections which mere partially calcified [49]. In this case, the underlying cause was shown to be filariasis which had been transmitted from the mother [49].

Other mode of transmissions including blood transfusionand vector transmission are more common for neonatal filariasis.

REFERENCES

[1] Casadevall A, Pirofski LA. Host-pathogen interactions: redefining the basic concepts of virulence and pathogenicity. *Infect Immun.* 1999; 67:3703-13.

[2] Casadevall A, Pirofski LA. Host-pathogen interactions: basic concepts of microbial commensalism, colonization, infection, and disease. *Infect Immun.* 2000; 68:6511-8.

[3] Wiwanitkit V. HIV transmission from mother to child: an aspect on the placenta barrier at the nano-level. *Aust N Z J Obstet Gynaecol.* 2005; 45:539-40.

[4] Wernsdorfer G, Wernsdorfer WH. Malaria at the turn from the 2nd to the 3rd millenium. *Wien. Klin. Wochenschr.* 2003; 115 Suppl 3: 2-9.

[5] Cot M, Deloron P. Malaria during pregnancy: consequences and interventional perspectives. *Med. Trop. (Mars).* 2003; 63: 369-80.

[6] Okoko BJ, Enwere G, Ota MO. The epidemiology and consequences of maternal malaria: a review of immunological basis. *Acta Trop.* 2003; 87: 193-205.

[7] Marques HH, Vallada MG, Sakane PT, Boulos M. Congenital Malaria. Case reports and a brief review of literature. *J Pediatr (Rio J).* 1996; 72: 103-5.

[8] Wiwanitkit V. Congenital malaria in Thailand, an appraisal of previous cases. *Pediatr Int.* 2006 Dec;48(6):562-5.

[9] Ahmed A, Cerilli LA, Sanchez PJ. Congenital malaria in a preterm neonate: case report and review of the literature. *Am J Perinatol.* 1998; 15: 19-22.

[10] Cichocka A, Skotarczak B. Babesosis--difficulty of diagnosis. *Wiad Parazytol.* 2001;47:527-33.

[11] Babesia research. Available on www.vetmed.ucdavis.edu/VBDP/BABESIA.HTM

[12] Allred DR, Al-Khedery B. Antigenic variation as an exploitable weakness of babesial parasites. *Vet Parasitol.* 2006; 138:50-60

[13] New DL, Quinn JB, Qureshi MZ, Sigler SJ. Vertically transmitted babesiosis. *J Pediatr.* 1997 Jul;131(1 Pt 1):163-4.

[14] Fox LM, Wingerter S, Ahmed A, Arnold A, Chou J, Rhein L, Levy O. Neonatal babesiosis: case report and review of the literature. *Pediatr Infect Dis J.* 2006 Feb;25(2):169-73.

[15] Murray HW, Berman JD, Davies CR, Saravia NG. Advances in leishmaniasis. Lancet 2005; 366:1561-77

[16] Gallego M. Emerging parasitic zoonoses: leishmaniosis. *Rev Sci Tech.* 2004; 23:661-76.

[17] Yurdakul P. Immunopathogenesis of Leishmania infections. *Mikrobiyol Bul.* 2005; 39:363-81.

[18] Piscopo TV, Mallia AC. Leishmaniasis. *Postgrad Med J.* 2006; 82:649-57.

[19] Murray HW, Berman JD, Davies CR, Saravia NG. Advances in leishmaniasis. *Lancet.* 2005; 366:1561-77.

[20] Meinecke CK, Schottelius J, Oskam L, Fleischer B. Congenital transmission of visceral leishmaniasis (Kala Azar) from an asymptomatic mother to her child. *Pediatrics.* 1999; 104:e65.

[21] Figueiro-Filho EA, Duarte G, El-Beitune P, Quintana SM, Maia TL. Visceral leishmaniasis (kala-azar) and pregnancy. *Infect Dis Obstet Gynecol.* 2004; 12(1):31-40.

[22] Eltoum IA, Zijlstra EE, Ali MS, Ghalib HW, Satti MM, Eltoum B, el-Hassan AM. Congenital kala-azar and leishmaniasis in the placenta. *Am J Trop Med Hyg.* 1992 Jan;46(1):57-62.

[23] Dey A, Singh S. Transfusion transmitted leishmaniasis: a case report and review of literature. *Indian J Med Microbiol.* 2006 Jul;24(3):165-70.

[24] Velarde CN. Chagas disease in Peru: congenital transmission. *Rev Soc Bras Med Trop.* 2005; 38 Suppl 2:55-7.

[25] Mendoza Ticona CA, Cordova Benzaquen E, Ancca Juarez J, Saldana Diaz J, Torres Choque A, Velasquez Talavera R, de los Rios Alvarez J, Saldana Diaz J, Vega Chirinos S, Sanchez Perez R. The prevalence of Chagas' disease in puerperal women and congenital transmission in an endemic area of Peru. *Rev Panam Salud Publica.* 2005 Mar; 17(3):147-53.

[26] Sanchez Negrette O, Mora MC, Basombrio MA. High prevalence of congenital Trypanosoma cruzi infection and family clustering in Salta, Argentina. *Pediatrics.* 2005 Jun;115(6):e668-72.

[27] Luquetti AO, Ferreira AW, Oliveira RA, Tavares SB, Rassi A, Dias JC, Prata A. Congenital transmission of Trypanosoma cruzi in Brazil: estimation of prevalence based on preliminary data of national serological surveys in children under 5 years old and other sources. *Rev Soc Bras Med Trop.* 2005; 38 Suppl 2:24-6.

[28] Sosa-Estani S. Congenital transmission of Trypanosoma cruzi infection in Argentina. *Rev Soc Bras Med Trop.* 2005; 38 Suppl 2:29-32.

[29] Blanco SB, Segura EL, Gurtler RE. Control of congenital transmission of Trypanosoma cruzi in Argentina. *Medicina (B Aires).* 1999; 59 Suppl 2:138-42.

[30] Bittencourt AL. Possible risk factors for vertical transmission of Chagas' disease. *Rev Inst Med Trop Sao Paulo.* 1992 Sep-Oct; 34(5):403-8.

[31] Neto EC, Rubin R, Schulte J, Giugliani R. Newborn screening for congenital infectious diseases. *Emerg Infect Dis.* 2004 Jun; 10(6):1068-73.

[32] Dlugonska H. Toxoplasma gondii--intracellular parasite. *Wiad Parazytol.* 2002; 48:23-8.

[33] Dodds EM. Toxoplasmosis. *Curr Opin Ophthalmol.* 2006; 17:557-61.

[34] Toxoplasmosis. Available on http://www.stanford.edu/class/humbio103/ParaSites2006/Toxoplasmosis/epidemiology.h

[35] Kravetz JD, Federman DG. Kravetz JD, Federman DG. Toxoplasmosis in pregnancy. *Am J Med.* 2005; 118:212-6.

[36] Jones J, Lopez A, Wilson M. Congenital toxoplasmosis. *Am Fam Physician.* 2003; 67:2131-8.

[37] Bale JF Jr. Congenital infections. *Neurol Clin.* 2002; 20:1039-60, vii.

[38] Martin S. Congenital toxoplasmosis. *Neonatal Netw.* 2001; 20:23-30.

[39] Georgiev VS. Management of toxoplasmosis. *Drugs.* 1994; 48:179-88.

[40] Gandahusada S. Study on the prevalence of toxoplasmosis in Indonesia: a review. *Southeast Asian J Trop Med Public Health.* 1991; 22 Suppl:93-8

[41] Raeber PA, Biedermann K, Just M, Zuber P. Prevention of congenital toxoplasmosis in Europe. *Schweiz Med Wochenschr Suppl.* 1995; 65:96S-102S.

[42] Gonzalez-Gonzalez NL, Dulin E, Barroso F, Domenech E. Neonatal screening for congenital toxoplasmosis by IgM anti-Toxoplasma determination in dried blood from the heel. *Enferm Infecc Microbiol Clin.* 2006 Dec; 24(10):664-5.

[43] Gomez-Marin JE, Gonzalez MM, Montoya MT, Giraldo A, Castano JC. A newborn screening programme for congenital toxoplasmosis in the setting of a country with less income. *Arch Dis Child.* 2007 Jan; 92(1):88

[44] Paul M, Petersen E, Pawlowski ZS, Szczapa J. Neonatal screening for congenital toxoplasmosis in the Poznan region of Poland by analysis of Toxoplasma gondii-specific IgM antibodies eluted from filter paper blood spots. *Pediatr Infect Dis J.* 2000 Jan;19(1):30-6.

[45] Carvalheiro CG, Mussi-Pinhata MM, Yamamoto AY, De Souza CB, Maciel LM. Incidence of congenital toxoplasmosis estimated by neonatal screening: relevance of diagnostic confirmation in asymptomatic newborn infants. *Epidemiol Infect.* 2005 Jun;133(3):485-91.

[46] Signorell LM, Seitz D, Merkel S, Berger R, Rudin C. Cord blood screening for congenital toxoplasmosis in northwestern Switzerland, 1982-1999. *Pediatr Infect Dis J.* 2006 Feb;25(2):123-8.

[47] Berger R, Sturchler D, Rudin C. Cord blood screening for congenital toxoplasmosis: detection and treatment of asymptomatic newborns in Basel, Switzerland. *Scand J Infect Dis Suppl.* 1992; 84:46-50.

[48] Dirofilariasis Information. Available at http://www.diseasesdatabase.com/ddb31226.htm

[49] Fonticiella M, Lopez-Negrete L, Prieto A, Garcia-Hernandez JB, Orense M, Fernandez-Diego J, Gomez JL. Congenital intracranial filariasis: a case report. *Pediatr Radiol.* 1995; 25(3):171-2.

[50] Neves Hde A, Scaff LM. Congenital microfilaria; preliminary report. *Rev Bras Malariol Doencas Trop.* 1952 Oct; 4(4):415-25.

[51] Ufomadu GO, Sato Y, Takahashi H. Possible transplacental transmission of Onchocerca volvulus. *Trop Geogr Med.* 1990 Jan; 42(1):69-71.

Chapter 16

TWIN - TWIN TRANSFUSION SYNDROME

INTRODUCTION TO TWIN PREGNANCY

Basically, a pregnant human usually bear one child or fetus. In some special cases, there might be more than one fetus in utero. This is called multiple pregnancy in medicine. The condition that there are two fetus in the same utero is well-known as twin pregnancy [1]. Twin can be originated from monozygote or heterozygote. Artificial reproductive technologies have led to a pronounced rise in numbers of dizygotic and monozygotic twins [2]. Although spontaneous dizygotic twinning is clearly associated with increased concentration of follicle-stimulating hormone and ovulation of more than one egg, causes of monozygotic twinning remain illusive [2]. For monozygotic twin, the production of twins/multiplets in livestock animal can be achieved either by microsurgical bisection of embryos at the morular- or blastocyst stage, isolation and proliferation of blastomeres from early cleavage stages or nuclear transfer [3]. This process is also the basis for human homozygotic twin. Monozygotic twinning seems to represent an anomaly in itself, with an increased number of spontaneous abortions and structural congenital anomalies [3]. Both monozygotic and dizygotic twins have growth rates that slow at 30 weeks in utero and might be programmed both developmentally and biochemically earlier in pregnancy to have different responses at birth and after birth compared with singletons [3].

There are also other well-known varieties of twin such as conjoined twin. Regarding the age old question of fusion or fission, it is concluded that there is no known embryologic process by which conjoined twins can be formed by fission but firm evidence to support fusion in all cases [4]. Whether the fusion occurs between embryos on one embryonic disc or on two is of no consequence since they are all monovular [4]. Intact ectoderm will not fuse to intact ectoderm, and all seven types of conjoined twins are explained by seven possible sites of union in the early embryo [4]. Presently, it is believed that conjoined twinning occurs by the incomplete splitting of the embryonic axis and, with the exception of parasitic conjoined twins, all are symmetrical and "the same parts are always united to the same parts" [5]. Fusion of monozygotic twins is no longer believed to be the basis of conjoined twinning [5]. Accounts are provided of the anatomical features of each of the commonly encountered varieties [5]. The most well-known conjoined twin is the Siamese twin, In-Chan.

There is a higher incidence of perinatal mortality and morbidity in twins than in singleton pregnancies [6]. The main reason for this increase is the higher incidence of preterm delivery in twins [6]. There are special conditions unique to twins that also contribute to this increased perinatal morbidity and mortality [6]. These conditions include monoamniotic twins, congenital anomalies unique to twins include conjoined twins and acardia, intrauterine fetal demise, and twin-to-twin transfusion syndrome [6]. The estimation of the rates of monozygotic and dizygotic twin maternities usually follows Weinberg's differential rule [7-9]. According to this rule, the rate of dizygotic twinning is twice the rate of twin maternities in which the twins are of opposite sex [7]. The monozygotic twinning rate is the difference between the rates of same-sex and opposite-sex twin sets [7]. Weinberg's differential rule is implicitly based on the assumptions that the probability of a male equals the probability of a female and that the sexes in a dizygotic twin set are independent [7-8].

Since 1980, there has been a worldwide dramatic increase in multiple births [10]. This seems to be due to an increase in the age of reproduction, the use of ovulation induction, and the use of in vitro fertilization [10]. Scarce data suggest that each of these causes is responsible for about one-third of the problem, although quintuplets and more are almost invariably due to ovulation induction [10]. Multiple pregnancies must be considered a serious adverse outcome of assisted reproductive techniques [10-12]. The international rates of triplet or higher order pregnancies after assisted reproduction are 7.3% at conception, 6.5% before reduction and 3.85% at birth [13]. Primary prevention of multiple pregnancies is the solution [10-12]. The infertility specialists who can solve the infertility problem are usually shielded from the complications of multiple pregnancies [11]. If they were involved in the delivery and, more particularly in the care of multiple pregnancies (both financially and socially), their attitude would probably change. The medical centres should gradually reduce the mean number of embryos per transfer in terms of the cost:benefit ratio [11]. New developments in blastocyst culture, single embryo transfer, embryo cryopreservation and pre-implantation aneuploidy exclusion, should allow improvements in pregnancy rates without increasing multiple pregnancies [10-12].

Problem of Twin Pregnancy

Twin pregnancy is considered as a problematic pregnancy. It should also be accepted as a public health problem [14]. The problems from twin pregnancy can be classified as maternal and fetal problem.

A. Maternal Problem

Since there are more than one fetus in utero, the mother has to take more effort in her pregnancy care. Multiple pregnancy is a high-risk pregnancy since it is associated with increased perinatal morbidity and mortality [15]. In addition, almost every maternal and obstetrical problem occurs more frequently in multiple than in singleton pregnancies [15]. The maternal mortality rate was 35.8/100.000 live births in twin pregnancies while it was 99/100000 in triplet gestation [15]. The management of multiple pregnancies includes early diagnosis, meticulous follow-up, and early decrease of maternal activity [16]. Data on the prognosis of triplet pregnancies are of particular importance when the option of selective termination is considered [16]. The most common complication is preterm labor [16]. Rolett and Kiely said that sociodemographic characteristics had weaker effects on preterm birth among twins than among singletons [17]. The prematurity rate is 50% in twin, 95% in triplet and 100% in multiple pregnancy of higher order [16]. The perinatal mortality was 20 to 80 per 1,000 in twins and 40 to 250 per 1,000 in triplets [16].

In additional to preterm labor, there are also other maternal complications due to twin pregnancy. Acute polyhydramnios in monozygotic twin pregnancy causes severe maternal discomfort and carries a high risk of premature labor [18-19]. Obstructive renal failure due to an overdistended uterus is a very rare complication of pregnancy [18]. Most previously reported cases have involved twin gestations, the majority occurring in the presence of polyhydramnios [18]. Acute obstructive uropathy should be considered as a rare cause of acute renal failure even in cases with seemingly normal pregnancy-induced physiological urinary tract dilation [18]. To face up with the problem of polyhydramios, Radestad and Thomassen reported that amniotic taps were safe if the amniotic fluid was removed slowly under prophylactic tocolysis [19]. It gives symptomatic relief to the mother and may postpone labor until the gestational age of the twins is more compatible with survival [19]. The antepartum death of one twin is a rare obstetric complication [20]. The premature and neonatal death rates are high in the surviving twins [20]. Toxemia, fetal distress, abnormal presentation, and dystocia are also increased [20]. The consumptive coagulopathy imposes a potential risk of health on both mother and the surviving fetus or neonate [20-23]. Maternal disseminated intravascular coagulation (DIC) has been demonstrated without a concomitant fetal coagulation defect [20]. The "vanished" twin is sometimes recognized as a fetus papyraceous (compressus) incorporated into the placenta of the survivor [21-22]. For the surviving infants, DIC can also be seen [21]. Death of one twin later in pregnancy may have serious implications for the survivor, especially in cases of monochorionic twins [22]. Neurological damage is also common for surviving infants [21]. Liu et al said that the probable cause of neurological damage was either exsanguination into the dead twin fetus [21]. Fusi and Gordon found that the prognosis for a surviving dichorionic twin was relatively good, with immaturity the main hazard while monochorionic twin had a poor prognosis with a high frequency of neurological damage [24]. Jaw et al said that obstetricians should be familiar with the management of one fetal death in twin pregnancy, especially in those with monchorionic twins [25]. Wang et al proposed that the appropriate time for delivery might depend on the duration of persistent D-dimer in the maternal blood [26]. The long-term presence of D-dimer in the maternal serum may indicate a severe underlying thromboembolic complication in the surviving twin after intrauterine death of a monochorionic twin [26]. Due to the increased risks of morbidity in premature births, the benefit of early termination of pregnancy in order to protect against subsequent sequelae in the surviving twin is minor [26].

For twin pregnancy, Colla et al proposed that that a more careful medical and social assistance, preventive hospitalization, early recognition of the risk, constant monitoring for the optimal timing of birth, and lastly, qualified medical assistance during labour (expert gynecologist, trained obstetric staff) with other medical personnel (anesthetist, neonatal specialist) represent winning strategies to solve the problems arising during multiple pregnancies [27].

B. Fetal Problem

Fetal and perinatal mortality is high in the twin pregnancy. The anomaly is a common fetal problem. A well-known condition is acardiac twin. Acardiac twinning, earlier known as chorioangiopagus parasiticus, is the most extreme manifestation of this condition [28]. An acardiac twin is a rare complication of multifetal pregnancy, in the literature reported at an incidence of 1% of monochorionic twin pregnancies, about 1 of 35,000 pregnancies [28]. Coulam and Wright said that suggest the pathogenesis of acardia involves arterioarterial anastomosis of placental vessels with retrogade blood flow into the recipient twin and not primary arrest in cardiac development [28-30]. Ultrasonography has assumed increasing importance in prenatal diagnosis of congenital anomalies [30]. Without treatment, the perinatal mortality of the pump twin is about 50-70% [29]. The optimal management of acardiac twin pregnancies is controversial [29]. Management options include elective termination, observation with close antepartum surveillance (serial cardiotocography, ultrasonography and echocardiography) and surgical interventions [29]. Wong and Sepulveda recently suggested a new classification system based on prognostic factors, specifically the size and growth of the acardiac twin and the cardiovascular condition of the pump twin [31]. In cases with a large acardiac twin or rapid growth of the acardiac mass, we recommend prompt intervention [31]. Once treatment is indicated, the intrafetal approach to interrupt the vascular supply to the acardiac twin appears to be superior to cord occlusion techniques as it is simpler, safer and more effective [31]. The first line of treatment should be ultrasound-guided laser coagulation or radiofrequency ablation of the intrafetal vessels [31]. Alternative treatments include injection of absolute alcohol (5 mL) into the intra-abdominal umbilical artery [32]. Acephalus twin is another interesting anomaly.This condition is also associated with acardiac twin and usually called holocardius acephalus twin [33]. The association of chromosome anomaly with holoacardius acephalus, especially for a 45,X chromosome constitution is noted [34].

A rare fetal complication is twin embolization syndrome (TES), a complication of monozygotic twinning following in utero demise of the co-twin [35]. Passage of thromboplastic material into the circulation of the surviving twin results in ischemic structural defects of the central nervous system, gastrointestinal tract, and genitourinary system [35-36]. Epilepsy is common sequelae in surviving infant [36]. Because of poor outcome, prenatal sonographic diagnosis of TES may influence antenatal or neonatal management of the surviving monozygous twin [35]. Recognition of TES may permit accurate postnatal counseling of prognosis and recurrence risks [35].

Umbilical cord abnormality is another interesting complication. entanglement and knotting of the cords leading to intrauterine death of both (more often) or one twin [37]. In monoamniotic pregnancy there should be a look for real knots of umbilical cord in regular intervals. In such a case, if a knot is present, the pregnant woman had to be supervised by colour doppler sonography, to react immediately at first signs of hypoxia [38]. Abdominal delivery upon reaching fetal lung maturity in the case of known monoamniotic twins is widely suggested [39]. Hospital admission for fetal monitoring upon discovery of a cord entanglement at a viable gestation is also advocated [39].

During delivery, twin interlocking is another rare complication that has a high fetal mortality and morbidity rate [40-43]. The proper delivery management is necessary. Piekarski et al reported that neonatal outcome depended on the mode of delivery and fetal presentation in twin gestation while time interval between vaginal delivery of twins had no significant impact on neonatal outcome [44].

TWIN- TWIN TRANSFUSION SYNDROME

Twin - twin transfusion syndrome is an important problematic in twin. is a severe complication occurring in monochorionic twins, and untreated, causes high rates of mortality and morbidity [45]. In twin - twin transfusion syndrome, five consecutive stages of increasing severity can be distinguished, the first is the oligo-polyhydramnios sequence, the second anuria in the donor twin, the third abnormal flow waves in either twin and the fourth a hydropic recipient with finally fetal demise of either twin [45]. The importance of fetal echocardiograms in assessing prognosis and response to therapy is highlighted [45]. The details on pathogenesis, clinical manifestation, diagnosis and treatment of this syndrome will be further discussed.

A. Pathogenesis

Basically, the cardiovascular system of the fetus is physiologically different than the adult, mature system [46]. Unique characteristics of the myocardium and specific channels of blood flow differentitate the physiology of the fetus from the newborn. Conditions of increased preload and afterload in the fetus, such as sacrococcygeal teratoma and twin-twin transfusion syndrome, result in unique and complex pathophysiological states [46]. Twin - twin transfusion syndrome is diamniotic twins that results from unbalanced blood flow from one to the other in utero [47]. Generally, twin-twin transfusion develops in 10-20% of monochorionic twin pregnancies [48]. The underlying disturbance is an unbalanced anastomosis between the two fetuses on the placental surface [48]. The increased rate of functional heart disease among the recipient twins in these pregnancies is a model for the theory of fetal origins of adult health [47]. Potential mechanisms for heart disease include alterations in the hormonal environment within the fetal bodies, blood pressure-driven alterations in blood flow and blood vessel distensibility, abnormal differentiation of fetal myocardial cells and changes in coronary artery growth [47]. Gardiner reported that a period of haemodynamic imbalance gave rise to changes in a muscular conduit artery that persist at least into infancy and it seemed that by correcting the abnormal haemodynamics relatively soon after the disease process had had begun, the alterations in elasticity were prevented [49].

B. Clinical Manifestation

Considering the natural history, the perinatal survival of twin-twin transfusion syndrome pregnancies managed without in utero procedures is approximately 30% overall and 63% in the four most recent series when diagnosed at < or = 28 weeks [50]. The classical clinical manifestation of twin – twin transfusion syndrome in surviving infant is an imbalance newborn birth size. Clinically, the donor twin will be anemic [51] and small while the recipient will be big but usually has the volume overload. Hikino et al reported that morbidity, growth and development of twin-twin transfusion syndrome survivors attained comparable levels of weight-matched controls, despite the higher neonatal mortality and these results suggested that the early management of twin-twin transfusion syndrome was critical for refining the total outcome of the affected twins [52].

The effect of intertwine transfusion is of interest. Bajoria et al found that fetal erythropoetin concentrations were higher in the twin-twin transfusion syndrome than non-twin-twin transfusion syndrome twin pairs and were correlated with the degree of hypoxemia, however, erythropoietin concentrations were comparable between donor and recipient twins, perhaps due to similar production rather than inter-twin transfusion of blood [53]. Bajora et al also found that the total stainable liver iron was comparable between twin pairs in the twin-twin transfusion syndrome and non- twin-twin transfusion syndrome groups [54]. Of interest, their study fails to provide evidence of iron overload in the recipient and depletion in the donor twins and, thereby, questions the validity of the conventional theory of inter-twin transfusion as the cause of twin-twin transfusion syndrome [54]. Denbow et al recently found that a hematocrit discordancy of more than 15 % was found in only 25 p7er cent of twin pairs [55]. In addition, there were no significant inter twin differences in the remaining indices [55].

Concerning the cardiac disturbance, features of cardiac hypertrophy with signs of a prehydropic or hydropic state develop during fetal life in recipient twins in twin-twin transfusion syndrome [56]. This impairment is reversible with the resolution of the fluid imbalance or after delivery [56]. Clinical manifestations in utero range from mild to critical pulmonary stenosis or lethal cardiomyopathy [57]. This finding is confirmed by the autopsy study [58]. However, Simpson et al recently proposed that prenatal cardiac dysfunction was common in recipient twins and could be transient, progressive, or persistent beyond the neonatal period [59]. Although perinatal prognosis seems to be related to the severity of dysfunction when first diagnosed in utero, follow up in infancy is recommended in view of the possibility of progressive pulmonary stenosis [57].

C. Diagnosis

Early diagnosis of twin-twin transfusion syndrome is important for prompt treatment. Denbow et al suggested that suggest that fetal blood sampling does not have a role in establishing the diagnosis of twin-twin transfusion syndrome, although its role in determining the degree of hematocrit discordancy to assist in timing of delivery remains to be evaluated [55]. One of the most effective tool for diagnosis of twin-twin transfusion syndrome in utero is the ultrasonography [60]. Jones et al suggested that suggest that the twin transfusion syndrome could be diagnosed in a significant number (81%) of cases [61]. They proposed that a disparity in antenatal fetal weights, size difference between the two amniotic sacs and a single placenta were present in upto 81% of confirmed cases [61]. However, the finding of two separate umbilical cords with a disparity in the size or number of vessels was rare and evidence of hydrops in either fetus or findings of congestive cardiac failure in the recipient twin were uncommon [61].

D. Treatment

Treatment strategies for this condition have remained controversial, but two main approaches have been commonly used [62]. Serial, aggressive amnioreduction and fetoscopic laser photocoagulation of the chorionic plate vascular anastomoses at the intertwin membrane [62]. Using the former technique, survival rates of between 18 and 83% have been described [62]. However, 5-58% neurological morbidity has been demonstrated in the surviving infants treated by serial amnioreduction alone [62]. A systematic review of observational and randomized controlled studies, laser photocoagulation of chorionic plate vessels at the intertwin membrane seems to be more effective than serial amnioreduction in the treatment of twin-twin transfusion syndrome with less associated perinatal morbidity and mortality [63]. However, septostomy and selective feticide have not been robustly evaluated [63-64].

REFERENCES

[1] Marivate M, Norman RJ. Twins. *Clin Obstet Gynaecol.* 1982 Dec;9(3):723-43.

[2] Hall JG. Twinning. *Lancet.* 2003 Aug 30;362(9385):735-43.

[3] Reichelt B, Niemann H. Production of monozygotic multiple offspring in agricultural domestic animals. *Dtsch Tierarztl Wochenschr.* 1996 Aug-Sep;103(8-9):340-8.

[4] Spencer R. Conjoined twins: theoretical embryologic basis. *Teratology.* 1992 Jun;45(6):591-602.

[5] Kaufman MH. The embryology of conjoined twins. *Childs Nerv Syst.* 2004 Aug;20(8-9):508-25.

[6] D'Alton ME, Simpson LL. Syndromes in twins. *Semin Perinatol.* 1995 Oct;19(5):375-86.

[7] Fellman J, Eriksson AW. Weinberg's differential rule reconsidered. *Hum Biol.* 2006 Jun;78(3):253-75.

[8] Jame WH. The current status of Weinberg's differential rule. *Acta Genet Med Gemellol (Roma).* 1992; 41(1):33-42.

[9] Renkonen KO. Is Weinberg's differential rule defective? *Ann Hum Genet.* 1967 Jan;30(3):277-80.

[10] Cohen J, Jones HW Jr. How to avoid multiple pregnancies in assistive reproductive technologies. *Semin Reprod Med.* 2001 Sep;19(3):269-78.

[11] Gurgan T, Demirol A. Why and how should multiple pregnancies be prevented in assisted reproduction treatment programmes? *Reprod Biomed Online.* 2004 Aug;9(2):237-44.

[12] Wimalasundera RC, Trew G, Fisk NM. Reducing the incidence of twins and triplets. *Best Pract Res Clin Obstet Gynaecol.* 2003 Apr;17(2):309-29.

[13] Cohen J. How to avoid multiple pregnancies in assisted reproduction. *Hum Reprod.* 1998 Jun;13 Suppl 3:197-214

[14] Olivennes F. Epidemiology: is twin pregnancy a public health problem? The gynecologists point of view. *J Gynecol Obstet Biol Reprod (Paris).* 2002 Feb;31(1 Suppl):2S8-10.

[15] Dafallah SE, Yousif EM. A comparative study of twin and triplet pregnancy. *Saudi Med J.* 2004 Apr;25(4):502-6.

[16] Pons JC. Multiple pregnancies. *Rev Prat.* 1995 Sep 15;45(14):1742-7.

[17] Rolett A, Kiely JL. Maternal sociodemographic characteristics as risk factors for preterm birth in twins versus singletons. *Paediatr Perinat Epidemiol.* 2000 Jul;14(3):211-8.

[18] Chung PH, Abramowicz JS, Edgar DM, Sherer DM. Acute maternal obstructive renal failure in a twin gestation despite normal physiological pregnancy-induced urinary tract dilation. *Am J Perinatol.* 1994 May;11(3):242-4.

[19] Radestad A, Thomassen PA. Acute polyhydramnios in twin pregnancy. A retrospective study with special reference to therapeutic amniocentesis. *Acta Obstet Gynecol Scand.* 1990; 69(4):297-300.

[20] Enbom JA. Twin pregnancy with intrauterine death of one twin. *Am J Obstet Gynecol.* 1985 Jun 15;152(4):424-9.

[21] Liu S, Benirschke K, Scioscia AL, Mannino FL. Intrauterine death in multiple gestation. *Acta Genet Med Gemellol (Roma).* 1992;41(1):5-26.

[22] Benirschke K. Intrauterine death of a twin: mechanisms, implications for surviving twin, and placental pathology. *Semin Diagn P*athol. 1993 Aug;10(3):222-31.

[23] Lin SH, Han CP, Liou JJ, Lu CC. Intrauterine single fetal demise in a twin gestation. A case report. *Zhonghua Yi Xue Za Zhi (Taipei).* 1989 Jul;44(1):61-4.

[24] Fusi L, Gordon H. Twin pregnancy complicated by single intrauterine death. Problems and outcome with conservative management. *Br J Obstet Gynaecol.* 1990 Jun;97(6):511-6.

[25] Jaw CS, Li YT, Hsu KP, Yeh KC, Tu FC, Tsui MS. Twin pregnancy complicated by single intrauterine death. Report of six cases and literature review. *Zhonghua Yi Xue Za Zhi (Taipei).* 1993 Apr;51(4):309-13.

[26] Wang KC, Yuan CC, Chao HT, Chang SP, Yang ML, Hung JH, Wang PH. Brain-damaged survivors after intrauterine death of a monochorionic twin. *Zhonghua Yi Xue Za Zhi (Taipei).* 2000 Sep;63(9):673-8.

[27] Colla F, D'Addato F, Grio R. Delivery in multiple pregnancies. *Minerva Ginecol.* 2001 Apr;53(2):101-5.

[28] Sogaard K, Skibsted L, Brocks V. Acardiac twins: pathophysiology, diagnosis, outcome and treatment. Six cases and review of the literature. *Fetal Diagn Ther.* 1999 Jan-Feb;14(1):53-9.

[29] Chanthasenanont A, Pongrojpaw D. Acardiac twin. *J Med Assoc Thai.* 2005 Nov;88(11):1721-4.

[30] Coulam CB, Wright G. First trimester diagnosis of acardiac twins. *Early Pregnancy.* 2000 Oct;4(4):261-70.

[31] Wong AE, Sepulveda W. Acardiac anomaly: current issues in prenatal assessment and treatment. *Prenat Diagn.* 2005 Sep;25(9):796-806.

[32] Rao A, Sairam S, Shehata H. Intrauterine treatment for an acardiac twin with alcohol injection into the umbilical artery. *J Obstet Gynaecol Res.* 2002 Apr;28(2):76-9.

[33] Reuhland RG, O'Leary JA, Ferrell RE. The holoacardius acephalus twin: prenatal diagnosis. *Am J Perinatol.* 1986 Jan;3(1):33-4.

[34] Deacon JS, Machin GA, Martin JM, Nicholson S, Nwankwo DC, Wintemute R. Investigation of acephalus. *Am J Med Genet.* 1980;5(1):85-99.

[35] Patten RM, Mack LA, Nyberg DA, Filly RA. Twin embolization syndrome: prenatal sonographic detection and significance. *Radiology.* 1989 Dec;173(3):685-9.

[36] Kawamura T, Morioka T, Fukui K, Nishio S, Hikino S, Gondo KJ. Symmetrical hemispheric porencephalic cysts due to twin embolization syndrome: a case report. *No To Shinkei.* 2002 Aug;54(8):723-8.

[37] Grzesiak M, Hincz P, Bielak A, Gulczynska E, Wilczynski J. Umbilical cord entanglement in monoamniotic twin preganacy--case presentation and literature review. *Ginekol Pol.* 2006 Sep;77(9):720-5.

[38] Krussel JS, von Eckardstein S, Schwenzer T. Double umbilical cord knot in mono-amniotic twin pregnancy as the cause of intrauterine fetal death of both twins. *Zentralbl Gynako*l. 1994;116(8):497-9.

[39] Ritossa M, O'Loughlin J. Monoamniotic twin pregnancy and cord entanglement: a clinical dilemma. *Aust N Z J Obstet Gynaecol.* 1996 Aug;36(3):309-12.

[40] Chia KV, Jayaratne T. Locked twins: a successful outcome. *Acta Obstet Gynecol Scand.* 1992 May;71(4):311-2.

[41] Fox RL, Nathanson HG, Tejani N, MAnn LI, Weiss RR. Interlocking twins. Experience with four cases and suggested management. *Obstet Gynecol.* 1975 Jul;46(1):53-7.

[42] Rachdi R, Fekih MA, Mouelhi C, Brahim H. Problems posed by the delivery of twin pregnancies. *Rev Fr Gynecol Obstet.* 1992 May;87(5):295-8.

[43] Unzeitig V, Uher M. Interlocking of twins. *Zentralbl Gynakol.* 1989; 111(22):1521-4.

[44] Piekarski P, Czajkowski K, Maj K, Milewczyk P. Neonatal outcome depending on the mode of delivery and fetal presentation in twin gestation. *Ginekol Pol.* 1997 Apr;68(4):187-92.

[45] van den Wijngaard JP, Ross MG, van Gemert MJ. Twin-Twin Transfusion Syndrome Modeling. *Ann N Y Acad Sci.* 2007 Mar 15;

[46] Rychik J. Fetal cardiovascular physiology. *Pediatr Cardiol.* 2004 May-Jun;25(3):201-9.

[47] Chescheir NC. Twin-to-twin transfusion syndrome: a model for the fetal origins of adult health. *Paediatr Perinat Epidemiol.* 2005 Jan;19 Suppl 1:32-6.

[48] Ek S, Bui TH, Westgren M. Twin-twin transfusion syndrome--front line in fetal medicine. *Lakartidningen.* 2001 Aug 29;98(35):3666-7, 3670-1.

[49] Gardiner HM. Early changes in vascular dynamics in relation to twin-twin transfusion syndrome. *Twin Res.* 2001 Oct;4(5):371-7.

[50] Berghella V, Kaufmann M. Natural history of twin-twin transfusion syndrome. *J Reprod Med.* 2001 May;46(5):480-4.

[51] Gill FM, Schwartz E. Anemia in early infancy. *Pediatr Clin North Am.* 1972 Nov;19(4):841-53.

[52] Hikino S, Ohga S, Kanda T, Nakashima T, Yamamoto J, Nakayama H, Nakano H, Hara T. Long-term outcome of infants with twin-to-twin transfusion syndrome. *Fetal Diagn Ther.* 2007; 22(1):68-74.

[53] Bajoria R, Ward S, Sooranna SR. Erythropoietin in monochorionic twin pregnancies in relation to twin--twin transfusion syndrome. *Hum Reprod.* 2001 Mar;16(3):574-80.

[54] Bajoria R, Lazda EJ, Ward S, Sooranna SR. Iron metabolism in monochorionic twin pregnancies in relation to twin--twin transfusion syndrome. *Hum Reprod.* 2001 Mar;16(3):567-73.

[55] Denbow M, Fogliani R, Kyle P, Letsky E, Nicolini U, Fisk N. Haematological indices at fetal blood sampling in monochorionic pregnancies complicated by feto-fetal transfusion syndrome. *Prenat Diagn.* 1998 Sep;18(9):941-6.

[56] Fesslova V, Villa L, Nava S, Mosca F, Nicolini U. Fetal and neonatal echocardiographic findings in twin-twin transfusion syndrome. *Am J Obstet Gynecol.* 1998 Oct;179(4):1056-62.

[57] Zosmer N, Bajoria R, Weiner E, Rigby M, Vaughan J, Fisk NM. Clinical and echographic features of in utero cardiac dysfunction in the recipient twin in twin-twin transfusion syndrome. *Br Heart J.* 1994 Jul;72(1):74-9.

[58] Bendon RW. Twin transfusion: pathological studies of the monochorionic placenta in liveborn twins and of the perinatal autopsy in monochorionic twin pairs. *Pediatr Pathol Lab Med.* 1995 May-Jun;15(3):363-76.

[59] Bendon RW. Cardiac dysfunction in twin-twin transfusion syndrome: a prospective, longitudinal study. *Obstet Gynecol.* 1998 Oct;92(4 Pt 1):557-62.

[60] Snijders R. First-trimester ultrasound. *Clin Perinatol.* 2001 Jun;28(2):333-52, viii.

[61] Jones JM, Sbarra AJ, Cetrulo CL. Twin transfusion syndrome: reassessment of ultrasound diagnosis. *J Reprod Med.* 1996 Jan;41(1):11-4.

[62] Duncan KR. Twin-to-twin transfusion: update on management options and outcomes. *Curr Opin Obstet Gynecol.* 2005 Dec;17(6):618-22.

[63] Fox C, Kilby MD, Khan KS. Contemporary treatments for twin-twin transfusion syndrome. *Obstet Gynecol.* 2005 Jun;105(6):1469-77.

[64] Roberts D, Neilson JP, Weindling AM. Interventions for the treatment of twin-twin transfusion syndrome. *Cochrane Database Syst Rev.* 2001; (1):CD002073.

Chapter 17

NEONATAL COAGULATION PROBLEM

INTRODUCTION TO COAGULATION DEFECT IN NEONATAL

Basically, successful blood stop must be composed of three basic effective components: good blood coagulation factor system, good platelet and good vascular structure. When there is an injury to the blood vessel, internal or external, the vessel firstly response by vasoconstriction. Then the coagulation cascade will start and process to finalize in fibrin network and platelet will go to accumulate at the injure size to get the complete blood stop process [1]. If there is any error in any basic component in any process, there will be a failure in blood stopping. On the other hand, there is a balance system to the coagulation process, the fibrinloytic system. If there is a defect in the balance system, the thrombotic disorder can also be detected. Thrombosis risk is multifactorial, with interaction of hereditary risk factors and acquired environmental and clinical conditions [2]. Newborns are at particular risk for thrombotic emergencies secondary to the unique properties of their hemostatic system, influences of the maternal-fetal environment, and perinatal complications and interventions [2]. The neonatal coagulation problem will be presented in this chapter.

PLATELET DEFECT IN THE NEONATE

Platelet defect in either quantity or quality can result in unsuccessful hemostasis. Platelet defect in neonate can also be seen. Basically, neonatal platelets are less reactive than adult platelets to physiological agonists in whole blood, as determined by the activation-induced increase in the platelet surface expression of P-selectin and the glycoprotein (GP) IIb-IIIa complex and by the activation-induced decrease in the platelet surface expression of the GPIb-IX complex [3]. Michelson et al suggested that the mechanism of neonatal platelet hyporeactivity is, at least in part, a relative defect in a common signal transduction pathway [3]. For the quantitative defect, abnormal low platelet or thrombocytopenia can be seen. Basically, thrombocytopenia is generally known in its most severe form as acquired immunologic disease [4]. However the frequency of neonatal thrombocytopenia in all newborns (< 150 x 10(9)/L) has been estimated at 1-4%. eonatal thrombocytopenia is a common clinical problem [4-6]. The majority of episodes are early-onset thrombocytopenias due to impaired fetal megakaryocytopoiesis associated with placental insufficiency; the commonest causes of severe early-onset thrombocytopenia are immune thrombocytopenias, congenital infections, and asphyxia [5]. However, in some cases thrombocytopenia is constitutional and may or may not be associated with thrombocytopathy [4]. The affected cases are characterized by the absence of significant bleeding disorders, stable thrombocyte counts higher than 50 x 10(9)/l, platelet macrocytosis, normal platelet function, normal or never increased presence of megakaryocytes, and rarely positive immunological abnormalities [4]. In all cases, platelet life span clearly indicated a defect of production with destruction linked to the ageing population (more than 7 days) and no abnormal sequestration in the spleen or liver [4]. By contrast, about 90% of cases of severe thrombocytopenia presenting after the first few days of life are due to late-onset bacterial sepsis, necrotizing enterocolitis, or both. Although clinically stable neonates tolerate relatively low platelet counts without significant risk of hemorrhage, ill or clinically unstable neonates with profound thrombocytopenia often have a poor outcome [5].

Concerning the immune thrombocytopenia, neonatal immune thrombocytopenia due to the transplacental passage of maternal antiplatelet IgG is a transient passive disease in an otherwise healthy newborn [6]. Indeed, the allo-immune thrombocytopenias are the major cause of severe thrombocytopenia in the fetus and the neonate [7]. The frequency of this affection has been evaluated to be 1 out of 800 to 1000 live births [7]. Autoimmune thrombocytopenic purpura in pregnant women can induce moderate or severe thrombocytopenia in the foetus or the newborn whatever the mother's disease status [6]. Fetal thrombocytopenia can occur as early as 20 weeks of gestation [6]. Heparin-induced thrombocytopenia (HIT), an immune-mediated response to heparin administration, has been recognized in adults for some time, but only recently recognized in neonates and children [8]. The incidence of HIT Type II is 2-5 percent in adults on heparin products and may be as high in neonates and children. The mortality rate from HIT in newborns is unknown but should be high [8]. l. The cardinal sign of HIT is a drop in platelet count by 50 percent or platelet counts below 70,000-100,000/mm^3 within five to ten days after the first exposure to heparin [8]. Treatment is immediate cessation of all heparin therapy and initiation of alternative anticoagulants, especially the direct thrombin inhibitors lepirudin and argatroban [8]. The major risk of severe thrombocytopenia is intracranial hemorrhage eading to death or neurological impairment [6]. Generally, an incidence of intracranial hemorrhage ICH in the neonatal period is 10-20%, and the autoimmune form with an incidence of only 1% [9]. Lopez-Lafuente et al suggested that cranial ecographic studies should be done in all newborn babies with immune thrombocytopenia even when no neurological disorder was seen [19]. They noted that an early diagnosis and suitable treatment might help to reduce the neurological sequelae [9]. Lopez-Lafuente et al also proposed that the neurological complications due to intraparenchymatous hemorrhage and visual sequelae were frequent [9].

Infection is also another important cause of thrombocytopenia in newborn. Bacterial sepsis is well-known to be the cause of neonatal thrombocytopenia [10-11]. The very low birth weight infant is the most high risk group. Common complications of sepsis in very low birth weight infants include anemia, thrombocytopenia, bleeding and multi-organ failure [10].

Strategies aimed at prevention, such as limiting the excessive use of broad-spectrum empiric antibiotics and the periodic review and continuous reinforcement of infection control policies will help decrease the mortality and morbidity associated with nosocomial infection in the very low birth weight infant [10]. There are important common infections relating to thrombocytopenia in the neonate that should be mentioned. Cytomegalovirus (CMV) is a common problematic infection and accepted as a member of TORCG agents that can be transmitted transplacentally. Basically, CMV is one of the Herpesviridae, known for their potential for latency and reactivation. The sequelae of fetal infection are diverse: chronic stage of early fetal infection with brain anomalies, symptomatic late fetal infection with hepatitis and thrombocytopenia and asymptomatic infection [12]. Neonatal adenovirus infection is another important infection-related cause of thrombocytopenia. Adenovirus infection in neonate is frequently disseminated and generally fatal, should be considered in the differential diagnosis of neonatal sepsis and pneumonia [13]. Common clinical findings includ lethargy, fever or hypothermia, anorexia, apnea, hepatomegaly, bleeding, and progressive pneumonia [13]. Thrombocytopenia, coagulopathy, and hepatitis are typical laboratory manifestations [13].

Necrotizing enterocolitis can be another important cause of neonatal thrombocytopenia. Necrotizing enterocolitis is the most common gastrointestinal emergency of the neonate, affecting 5-10% of infants [14]. Widely accepted risk factors include prematurity, enteral feeds, bacterial colonization and mucosal injury [14]. The activation of the cytokine cascade, in part by bacterial ligands, appears to play a key role in mucosal injury [14]. Severe thrombocytopenia frequently accompanies advanced necrotizing enterocoliti. In premature infants with severe thrombocytopenia, despite a paucity of evidence to support the practice, platelet transfusions are commonly used to maintain arbitrary levels of platelet counts in an effort to prevent hemorrhage. However, platelet transfusions contain a variety of bioactive factors, including platelet activating factor, which can augment systemic inflammatory processes [15].

Considering the impairment of platelet quality, it is usually accompanied with decreased platelet quantity. The good example is the dengue infection. Dengue infection is a mosquito borne infection that is endemic in many tropical countries. This infection manifests as a common triad: hemoconcentration, thrombocytopenia and high fever. It should be noted that dengue infection can be seen in the neonate [16]. In addition, the congenital dengue infection is also reported [16]. Wiwanitkit proposed that platelet CD61 might have an important role in causing hemorrhagic complication in dengue infection [17]. For the underlying of pathogenesis of thrombocytopenia, the immune mimicking theory is a widely mentioned [16-17]. The principal aim in the management of the affected infants with thrombocytopenia is to prevent the deleterious consequences of severe thrombocytopenia [6]. Supportive treatment should be effectively administered. Platelet transfusion might be needed [4-6]. If there is an identified cause such as infection, the physician should also get rid of the primary root.

Vascular Defect in the Neonate

Vascular defect that can lead to bleeding presentation is not common. A condition that relating to vascular that can lead to bleeding in pediatric population is vitamin C deficiency. Physiologically, bitamin C is an important vitamin for the hemostasis process. The main action of vitamin C in the hemostasis process is mainly on the vascular component. Vitamin C deficiency can lead to the most well-known vitamin deficiency disease, scurvy. Scurvy and periodontitis both manifest gingival bleeding but constitute separate entities [18]. Defective collagen in scurvy reflects many symptoms emanating from deficient vitamin C physiology [18]. Its prominent clinical features are lethargy; purpuric lesions, especially affecting the legs; myalgia; and, in advancing disease, bleeding from the gums with little provocation [19]. Common misdiagnoses are vasculitis, blood dyscrasias, and ulcerative gingivitis [22]. Untreated, scurvy is inevitably fatal as a result of infection or sudden death [19]. Fortunately, individuals with scurvy, even those with advanced disease, respond favorably to administration of vitamin C [19]. Recently, Ratanachu-Ek et al studied 28 cases of scurvy [20]. According to this study, they concluded that vitamin C deficiency was found in the children's intake of small amounts or no vegetables and fruits together with UHT-milk [20]. They noted that frequent manifestations of scurvy were limping and inability to walk and pain in the lower limbs and response to vitamin C treatment was dramatic [20]. Neonatal scurvy is an important neonate nutritional problem [21-22]. There are many possible unwanted complications of neonatal scurvy including epiphyseo-metaphyseal cupping [22] and spinal change [23].

Coagulation Defect in the Neonate

Coagulation defect that can lead to bleeding presentation is common. There are many congenital defects of coagulation factor system. The most well-known is hemophilia. Hemophilia is one of the oldest known hereditary bleeding disorder. There are two main types of hemophilia, A and B (Christmas Disease). Low levels or complete missing of a blood protein essential for clotting causes both types. Patients with hemophilia A lack the blood clotting protein, factor VIII, and those with hemophilia B lack factor IX [24]. The severity of hemophilia is usually related to the amount of the clotting factor in the blood [24]. About 70% of hemophilia patients have less than one percent of the normal amount and, therefore, have severe hemophilia [24]. A small increase in the blood level of the clotting factor, up to five percent of normal, results in mild hemophilia with rare bleeding except after injuries or surgery [24]. In people with hemophilia, blood does not clot as it should because it is missing or has low levels of one of these clotting factors [25]. If blood doesn't clot as quickly or as well as it should, then: a) heavy blood loss can occur, b) body organs and tissues can be injured, and c) these conditions can result in permanent damage or death [25]. Sometimes people with hemophilia need infusions of a clotting factor or factors to stop bleeding [25]. In the presence of a family history of haemophilia optimal management requires close co-operation between three individual specialist groups - obstetricians, haematologists and neonatologists, who each have an important role to play in ensuring a safe outcome for these infants [26].

Hemophilia A is caused by partial or complete depletion of factor VIII. In general, hemophilia is more common than hemophilia B [24-25]. Technologies in molecular biology have greatly advanced the knowledge regarding the origin of haemophilia A and the physiology of the factor VIII protein [27]. It is an X-linked recessive bleeding disorder affecting one in 10,000 males [28]. Prevalence of the haemophilia gene in the general population has increased recently due to advances in treatment, which has resulted in reproductive fitness among heamophiliacs [28]. A variety of different mutations in the factor VIII gene have been identified and their effects on the factor VIII protein described [26]. Basically, Factor VIII gene is very large with 26 exons [28]. Defects in this gene result in the deficiency of factor VIII molecule [28]. It has been shown that the frequency of haemophilia A is due to a high mutation rate predominantly in male germ cells [28]. A significant proportion is originating de novo in early embryogenesis from somatic mutations, a finding that has implications for genetic counseling [28]. Most recently it has been shown that FVIII clearance from the circulation is mediated by the low-density lipoprotein receptor-related protein (LRP) and cell-surface heparan sulphate proteoglycans (HSPGs) [28]. With the advent of recent advances in the molecular biology, it is possible to identify the multiple molecular defects such as point mutations, premature stop codons, deletions, and inversions etc in the FVIII gene in patients with haemophilia [29]. Nowadays the use of polymerase chain reaction (PCR)-based linkage analysis and direct mutation detection in the chorionic villus sample obtained at 10-12 weeks of gestation has significantly improved the prenatal diagnosis of haemophilia [28]. Southern blot analysis successfully detected a carrier in a hemophilia family for which no patient was available [29]. It should be noted that major organ bleeding in severe haemophilia A in the newborn period is rare, and this unusual complication is not well recognized [30]. Failure to recognize that the bleeding is due to a bleeding disorder, particularly in the absence of a family history, may lead to delay in appropriate management [30].

Haemophilia B, an X-linked recessive bleeding disorder due to factor IX (FIX) deficiency, has an incidence of about 1:30,000 live male births. The factor 9 (F9) gene was mapped on Xq27.1. Several factor IX deficiency disorders are reported [31]. The one known as hemophilia Bm variant, factor IXHilo, is the new deficiency first described in Europe [32]. Pathophysiologically, a point mutation that resulted in the substitution of a glutamine (CAG) for an arginine (CGG) at amino acid 180 is found in exon VI of the factor IX gene (G----A at nucleotide 20519) [32]. This mutation alters the carboxy terminal cleavage site for the activation peptide at Arg180-Val181 [32]. For hemophilia B, it is diagnosed from prothrombin time, activated partial thromboplastin time, and factor IX levels [33]. Similar to hemophilia A, several molecular tools are used for diagnosis of hemophilia B. The recent progress in the uses of factor IX gene probes in clinical diagnosis of hemophilia B carriers, as well as their use for analyzing the structural gene abnormalities that are responsible for the disease should be noted [34]. Generally, carrier females are usually asymptomatic and must be identified only with molecular analysis [33]. Linkage analysis of factor 9 polymorphisms is rapid and inexpensive but limited by non-informative families, recombinant events, and the high incidence of germline mutations; thus, various procedures have been used for the direct scan of factor 9 mutations [33]. A novel denaturing high performance liquid chromatographic procedure to scan the factor 9 gene is also launched [33]. However, the complicated technology is lack in the developing countries. The basic classical test is still needed in these settings.

The clinical manifestations of hemophilia depend upon both age and the severity of the factor VIII or IX deficiency [35]. Laboratory tests include platelet count, prothrombin time, partial thromboplastin time, and bleeding time [35]. the transfusion is an important tool for treatment of the patients with hemophilia. The clotting factor can be prepared from the donated blood. The problem on finding of blood donor and donor selection should be mentioned. In addition, the problem of blood borne infection in the present day should be stated. Human immunodeficiency virus (HIV) and hepatitis C virus (HCV) in the blood supply are the important problematic blood borne transmitted diseases. The risk of pathogen transmission via clotting factor therapies has been reduced over the last two decades through the development of effective and progressively more sensitive pathogen screening and inactivation methods and the introduction of recombinant clotting factors for hemophilia, beginning with recombinant factor VIII in 1992 [36]. However, new understanding about the potential for transmission of an emerging infectious agent through blood and blood products has renewed concerns about vulnerabilities that remain in plasma-derived and some recombinant clotting therapies that still use plasma components during some stages of the manufacturing process [36].

In addition to congenital coagulation factor defect, there are also other acquired conditions in neonate. One of the well-known conditions is disseminated intravascular coagulopathy (DIC). This condition also affects the platelet. Quick action is necessary to determine the cause of bleeding, which determines how the infant will be treated [37]. DIC is usually an uncontrolled, simultaneous bleeding and clotting occurring as a secondary disorder in sick neonates [37]. The newborn infant is particularly susceptible to DIC because of several handicaps, such as physiological hypofunction of anticoagulant and fibrinolytic systems, an underdeveloped capacity in the reticuloendothelial system and a tendency to develop acidosis, hypothermia, hypoxia and shock [38]. Although some criteria have been reported for the diagnosis of DIC in adults, based on clinical and laboratory findings, these are not necessarily applicable to the diagnosis of DIC in newborn infants [38]. This is because a large blood sample is required, a long period of time is necessary for assay and difference in several coagulation and fibrinolysis factors exist between newborn infants and adults [38]. Shirahata et al indicated that the scoring system for platelet counts in diagnostic criteria of DIC in newborn infants was applicable to the diagnosis of DIC in very low birth weight infants, however, the scoring systems for fibrinogen and D-dimer were not usable for the diagnostic criteria of DIC in very low birth weight infants since fibrinogen and D-dimer concentrations in very low birth weight infants without DIC were lower than those in non-DIC neonates whose birth weights were above 1500 grams [39]. Knowledge of the complex physiologic mechanisms at work to maintain hemostasis contributes to the proper nursing care of infants at risk for DIC and better outcomes [37].

Thrombohemostatic Defect in the Neonate

Thrombohemostatic disorder is an important hematological disorder in neonatology. Venous thromboembolism is an increasingly recognised problem in pediatric practice, particularly in the context of tertiary care pediatric services [40]. Several thrombohemostatic disoders are described for the neonates. Neonatal cerebrovenous sinus thrombosis is extremely rare, however it is a devastating condition and one needs to be aware of this condition to diagnose it [41]. Gestational or delivery complications or risk factors and comorbid conditions such as dehydration, sepsis, and cardiac defects are common for neonatal cerebrovenous sinus thrombosis [42]. Fitzgerald et al proposed that the presentation of neonatal SVT was often nonspecific, the diagnosis could be difficult to make, treatment beyond supportive care was rarely used, and outcomes can be severe [42]. Concerning the arterial thromboembolism, perinatal stroke has become increasingly recognized, but the incidence is probably underestimated because of variation in the presentation, evaluation, and diagnosis [43]. Perinatal arterial ischemic stroke in infants is associated with several independent maternal risk factors [44-45]. Maternal conditions that have been associated with perinatal stroke in the fetus include prothrombotic disorders, cocaine abuse, and placental complications such as chorioamnionitis and placental vasculopathy [44]. In many cases, the placenta is suspected to be the underlying embolic source for perinatal stroke, although data on placental pathology is often lacking [44]. During the delivery process, an infant may develop a cervical arterial dissection that leads to stroke [44]. Several conditions in the neonatal period predispose to perinatal stroke including prothrombotic disorders, congenital heart disease, meningitis, and systemic infection [44]. Based on estimates from population-based studies of infants with seizures, perinatal stroke occurs in approximately 1 in 4000 term births [43]. Perinatal stroke may present with neonatal seizures during the first weeks of life or may be asymptomatic until months later when the infant is first noted to have pathological handedness [43]. Perinatal stroke underlies an important share of congenital hemiplegic cerebral palsy, and probably some spastic quadriplegic cerebral palsy and seizure disorders [46]. The outcome of perinatal stroke is variable and depends on severity, anatomic localization, and other factors not yet well clarified [44].

REFERENCES

[1] Goldenberg NA, Manco-Johnson MJ. Pediatric hemostasis and use of plasma components. *Best Pract Res Clin Haematol.* 2006; 19(1):143-55.

[2] Thornburg C, Pipe S. Neonatal thromboembolic emergencies. *Semin Fetal Neonatal Med.* 2006 Jun;11(3):198-206.

[3] Michelson AD. Platelet function in the newborn. *Semin Thromb Hemost.* 1998; 24(6):507-12.

[4] Najean Y, Lecompte T. Hereditary thrombocytopenias in childhood. *Semin Thromb Hemost.* 1995; 21(3):294-304.

[5] Roberts IA, Murray NA. Neonatal thrombocytopenia. *Curr Hematol Rep.* 2006 Mar;5(1):55-63.

[6] Kaplan C. Immune thrombocytopenia in the foetus and the newborn: diagnosis and therapy. *Transfus Clin Biol.* 2001 Jun;8(3):311-4.

[7] Kaplan C. Fetal/neonatal allo-immune thrombocytopenias: the unsolved questions. *Transfus Clin Biol.* 2005 Jun;12(2):131-4.

[8] Martchenke J, Boshkov L. Heparin-induced thrombocytopenia in neonates. *Neonatal Netw.* 2005 Sep-Oct;24(5):33-7.

[9] Lopez-Lafuente A, Campistol J, Toll MT, Iriondo M. Perinatal intracranial hemorrhage due to immune thrombocytopenia. *Rev Neurol.* 1999 Nov 16-30;29(10):917-22.

[10] Trotman H, Bell Y. Neonatal sepsis in very low birthweight infants at the University Hospital of the West indies. *West Indian Med J.* 2006 Jun;55(3):165-9.

[11] Boyer KM. Diagnosis of neonatal sepsis. *Mead Johnson Symp Perinat Dev Med.* 1982; (21):40-6.

[12] Lagasse N, Dhooge I, Govaert P. Congenital CMV-infection and hearing loss. *Acta Otorhinolaryngol Belg.* 2000; 54(4):431-6.

[13] Abzug MJ, Levin MJ. Neonatal adenovirus infection: four patients and review of the literature. *Pediatrics.* 1991 Jun;87(6):890-6.

[14] Gibbs K, Lin J, Holzman IR. Necrotising enterocolitis: the state of the science. *Indian J Pediatr.* 2007 Jan;74(1):67-72.

[15] Fernandes CJ, O'Donovan DJ. Platelet transfusions in infants with necrotizing enterocolitis. *Curr Hematol Rep.* 2006 Mar;5(1):76-81.

[16] Wiwanitkit V. Dengue haemorrhagic fever in pregnancy: Appraisal on Thai cases. *J Vector Borne Dis.* 2006 Dec;43(4):203-5.

[17] Wiwanitkit V. Platelet CD61 might have an important role in causing hemorrhagic complication in dengue infection. *Clin Appl Thromb Hemost.* 2005 Jan;11(1):112.

[18] Touyz LZ. Vitamin C, oral scurvy and periodontal disease. *S Afr Med J.* 1984 May 26;65(21):838-42.

[19] Pimentel L. Scurvy: historical review and current diagnostic approach. *Am J Emerg Med.* 2003 Jul;21(4):328-32.

[20] Ratanachu-Ek S, Sukswai P, Jeerathanyasakun Y, Wongtapradit L. Scurvy in pediatric patients: a review of 28 cases. *J Med Assoc Thai.* 2003 Aug;86 Suppl 3:S734-40.

[21] Hirsch M, Mogle P, Barkli Y. Neonatal scurvy: report of a case. *Pediatr Radiol.* 1976 Aug 20;4(4):251-3.

[22] Sprogue PL.Epiphyseo-metaphyseal cupping following infantile scurvy. *Pediatr Radiol.* 1976 Feb 13;4(2):122-3.

[23] Maclean AD. Spinal changes in a case of infantile scurvy. *Br J Radiol.* 1968 May;41(485):385-7.

[24] Hemophilia. Available at http://www.medceu.com/tests/hemophilia.htm

[25] Hemophilia. Available at http://www.nhlbi.nih.gov/health/dci/Diseases/hemophilia/hemophilia_what.html

[26] Chlamers EA. Haemophilia and the newborn. *Blood Rev.* 2004 Jun;18(2):85-92.

[27] Oldenburg J, Ananyeva NM, Saenko EL. Molecular basis of haemophilia A. *Haemophilia.* 2004 Oct;10 Suppl 4:133-9.

[28] Saxena R, Mohanty S, Choudhry VP. Prenatal diagnosis of haemophilia. *Indian J Pediatr.* 1998 Sep-Oct;65(5):645-9.

[29] Fukuda K, Naka H, Morichika S, Shibata M, Tanaka I, Shima M, Yoshioka A. Inversions of the factor VIII gene in Japanese patients with severe hemophilia A. *Int J Hematol.* 2004 Apr;79(3):303-6.

[30] Hamilton M, French W, Rhymes N, Collins P. Liver haemorrhage in haemophilia--a case report and review of the literature. *Haemophilia.* 2006 Jul;12(4):441-3.

[31] Bowen DJ. Haemophilia A and haemophilia B: molecular insights. *Mol Pathol.* 2002; 55:127-44.

[32] Huang MN, Kasper CK, Roberts HR, Stafford DW, High KA. Molecular defect in factor IXHilo, a hemophilia Bm variant: Arg----Gln at the carboxyterminal cleavage site of the activation peptide. *Blood.* 1989; 73:718-21.

[33] Castaldo G, Nardiello P, Bellitti F, Santamaria R, Rocino A, Coppola A, di Minno G, Salvatore F. Haemophilia B: from molecular diagnosis to gene therapy. *Clin Chem Lab Med*. 2003 Apr;41(4):445-51.

[34] Tonimoto M. Factor IX molecular defects in diagnosing hemophilia B: a review. *Nippon Ketsueki Gakkai Zasshi.* 1989 Jul;52(4):811-5.

[35] Buchanan GR. Hemophilia. *Pediatr Clin North Am.* 1980 May;27(2):309-26.

[36] Pipe S. Consideration in hemophilia therapy selection. *Semin Hematol.* 2006 Apr;43(2 Suppl 3):S23-7.

[37] Keuhl J. Neonatal disseminated intravascular coagulation. *J Perinat Neonatal Nurs.* 1997 Dec;11(3):69-77.

[38] Shirahata A, Shirakawa Y. New approach to the diagnosis of disseminated intravascular coagulation in childhood. *Nippon Rinsho.* 1993 Jan;51(1):61-6.

[39] Shirahata A, Shirakawa Y, Murakami C. Diagnosis of DIC in very low birth weight infants. *Semin Thromb Hemost.* 1998; 24(5):467-71.

[40] Chalmers EA. Epidemiology of venous thromboembolism in neonates and children. *Thromb Res.* 2006; 118(1):3-12.

[41] Ibrahim HS. Cerebral venous sinus thrombosis in neonates. *J Pak Med Assoc.* 2006 Nov;56(11):535-7.

[42] Fitzgerald KC, Williams LS, Garg BP, Carvalho KS, Golomb MR. Cerebral sinovenous thrombosis in the neonate. *Arch Neurol.* 2006 Mar;63(3):405-9.

[43] Lynch JK, Nelson KB. Epidemiology of perinatal stroke. *Curr Opin Pediatr.* 2001 Dec;13(6):499-505.

[44] Wu YW, Lynch JK, Nelson KB. Perinatal arterial stroke: understanding mechanisms and outcomes. *Semin Neurol.* 2005 Dec;25(4):424-34.

[45] Lee J, Croen LA, Backstrand KH, Yoshida CK, Henning LH, Lindan C, Ferriero DM, Fullerton HJ, Barkovich AJ, Wu YW. Maternal and infant characteristics associated with perinatal arterial stroke in the infant. *JAMA.* 2005 Feb 9;293(6):723-9.

[46] Nelson KB, Lynch JK. Stroke in newborn infants. *Lancet Neurol.* 2004 Mar;3(3):150-8.

Chapter 18

NEONATAL HEMOCHROMATOSIS

IRON METABOLISM: AN OVERVIEW

Iron is one of the most important trace elements for human beings. Dietary heme is an important source of iron for the body which is taken up intact by the enterocyte [1]. Iron metabolism in mammals requires a complex and tightly regulated molecular network [2]. The classical view of iron metabolism has been challenged over the past ten years by the discovery of several new proteins, mostly Fe (II) iron transporters, enzymes with ferro-oxydase (hephaestin or ceruloplasmin) or ferri-reductase (Dcytb) activity or regulatory proteins like HFE and hepcidin [2]. Total body iron homeostasis is dependent upon carefully regulated absorption of dietary iron, thus these genes are of fundamental importance in understanding of pathophysiology of such common disorders as hereditary hemochromatosis and the anaemia of chronic diseases [3]. The hepatic peptide hepcidin plays a key role as a circulating hormone that regulates the absorption of dietary iron from the duodenum [3]. Other hepatic proteins essential for normal iron homeostasis, including HFE, transferrin receptor 2, and hemojuvelin, function at least in part, by modulating the expression of hepcidin [3]. The iron deficiency is an important nutritional disorder. Molecularly, overexpression of hepcidin results in iron-deficiency anemia in mice and hepcidin levels decrease in mice fed a low iron diet [4]. Hypochromic microcytic anemia can be the result of iron deficiency. A report from the World Health Organization estimates that 46% of the world's 5- to 14-year-old children are anemic [5]. In addition, 48% of the world's pregnant women are anemic [5]. A majority of these cases of anemia are due to iron deficiency [5].

However, the properties that make iron a necessity also make it potentially deleterious [6]. To avoid harm, iron homeostasis is achieved through iron transport, storage and regulatory proteins [6]. The functions of some of these molecules are well described, for example transferrin and transferrin receptor-1, whereas the roles of others, such as the transferrin homolog melanotransferrin, remain unclear [6]. Although the recent identification of several genes has extended our knowledge on the maintenance of body iron homeostasis, their tissue specific expression patterns and the underlying regulatory networks are poorly understood [7]. Ludwiczek et al suggested that the feed back regulation of duodenal iron absorption by hepcidin was impaired in genetic hemochromatosis [7]. This change may be linked to inappropriate iron sensing by the liver based on decreased TfR-2 expression, resulting in reduced circulating hepcidin levels and an inappropriate up-regulation of Dcytb driven iron absorption [6]. In addition, iron excretion/reabsorption by the kidneys may be altered, which may aggravate progressive iron overload [7]. In this chapter, the hemochromatosis in the neonate group will be focused.

Introduction to Hemochromatosis

Hemochromatosis is a common genetic condition and yet there are still a number of misperceptions surrounding the diagnosis and management of this condition [8]. Hemochromatosis affects both men and women [8]. Typical patients do not have alcoholism or viral hepatitis, and often have normal liver enzymes [8]. The spectrum of this disease is very wide. Hemochromatosis can be primary or secondary. For primary hemochromatosis, the heriditary hemochromatosis is the most well-known condition. A number of genetic disorders can result in the accumulation of excess iron in the body [9]. These causes of hereditary hemochromatosis include defects in genes encoding HFE, transferrin receptor 2, ferroportin, hepcidin, and hemojuvelin [9]. As previously mentioned, hepcidin plays important role in the molecular pathogenesis of hemochromatosis. Hepcidin is a cationic amphipathic peptide made in the liver, released into plasma and excreted in urine [10]. Hepcidin is the homeostatic regulator of intestinal iron absorption, iron recycling by macrophages, and iron mobilization from hepatic stores, but it is also markedly induced during infections and inflammation [10]. Under the influence of hepcidin, macrophages, hepatocytes, and enterocytes retain iron that would otherwise be released into plasma [10]. In concordance with this dual function its expression is modulated by systemic iron requirements and in response to infectious and inflammatory stimuli [11]. Furthermore, a deregulation of hepcidin may cause elevated intestinal iron absorption that hallmarks a group of frequent iron overload disorders, the hereditary hemochromatosis [11].

In addition to the primary hemochromatosis, secondary hemochromatosis can be seen in clinical practice. Basically, secondary iron overload constitutes a growing clinical problem, particularly in haematological diseases in which the improvements of life expectancy give the iron overload enough duration to play its own prognostic role [12]. Iron may accumulate by two ways: transfusion and digestive hyperabsorption which is proportional to erythroid plasma iron turnover [12]. However, the most common condition that can lead to the secondary hemochromatosis is the repeated hypertransfusion. Transfusion therapy for inherited anemias and acquired refractory anemias both improves the quality of life and prolongs survival [13]. However, a consequence of chronic transfusion therapy is secondary iron overload, which adversely affects the function of the heart, the liver and other organs [13]. Regular blood transfusions in thalassaemia and other chronic refractory anaemias can result in excessive iron deposition in tissues and organs [14]. This excess iron is toxic, resulting in tissue and organ damage and unless it is removed it can be fatal to those chronically transfused. Iron removal in transfusional iron overload is achieved using chelation therapy with the chelating drugs deferoxamine and deferiprone (L1) [14]. The introduction of the iron-chelating agent dramatically improved the life expectancy of these patients [15]. However, the very demanding nature of this treatment (subcutaneous, continuous infusion via a battery-operated portable pump) has been the motivation for attempts to develop alternative forms of treatment that would facilitate the patients' compliance [15].

HEREDIATARY HEMOCHROMATOSIS

A. Genetic Underlying

Hereditary hemochromatosis is a genetic metabolic disease characterized by increased intestinal iron absorption and progressive iron loading in the cells of various organs [16-17]. Human body iron homeostasis involves a number of complicated processes, some of which are not identified yet [16-17]. In recent years, the number of proteins implicated in iron homeostasis has increased dramatically, and genetic causes have apparently been identified for the major disorders associated with tissue iron overload [16]. The elucidation of the molecular pathways of iron transport through cells and its control has led to the understanding of various genetic iron-loading conditions [18]. Four types of inherited iron overload have been recognized: type 1, the most common form with an autosomal recessive inheritance, is associated with mutations in the HFE gene on chromosome 6; type 2 (juvenile hemochromatosis) is an autosomal recessive disorder with causative mutations identified in the HJV gene (subtype A) on chromosome 1 and the HAMP gene (subtype B) on chromosome 19; type 3 has also an autosomal recessive inheritance with mutations in the TfR2 gene on chromosome 3; type 4 is an autosomal dominant condition with heterozygous mutations in the ferroportin 1 gene on chromosome 2 [18]. The most common form of primary hemochromatosis is that caused by C282Y mutation of the HFE gene [19]. This mutation is most prevalent among Northern Europeans [19]. Although the frequency of the homozygous genotype is approximately 5 per 1000, the disease itself is quite rare because the clinical penetrance of the genotype is very low [19].

The availability of a facile treatment for hemochromatosis renders early diagnosis of iron overload syndromes mandatory, and in many instances genetic testing allows identification of individuals at risk of developing clinical disease before pathologic iron storage occurs [20]. Although most adult patients with hereditary iron overload are homozygous for the C282Y mutation of the HFE gene, an increasing number with hereditary iron storage have an HFE genotype not characteristic of the disease [20]. Heterozygosity for mutations in the gene encoding ferroportin 1 is probably the second most common genetic cause of hereditary iron storage in adults; here the primarily affected cell is the macrophage. Rare defects, including mutations in the transferrin receptor 2 gene, have also been identified in pedigrees affected with "non-HFE hemochromatosis [20]."

B. Pathogenesis

Recent advances in our understanding of iron metabolism, the identification of the gene responsible for hemochromatosis, and large epidemiologic studies have changed the diagnostic approach toward patients with hereditary hemochromatosis and other forms of iron overload [21]. The most common form of this disorder is HFE-related HH, nearly always caused by homozygosity for the C282Y mutation [22]. A substantial proportion of C282Y homozygotes do not develop clinically significant iron overload, suggesting roles for environmental factors and modifier genes in determining the phenotype [22]. Two major hypotheses have been proposed to explain the pathogenesis of HFE-related hereditary hemochromatosis: the hepcidin hypothesis and the duodenal crypt cell programming hypothesis [23]. Recent studies have demonstrated that the pathogenesis of nearly all forms of herediatary hemochromatosis involves inappropriately decreased expression of the iron-regulatory hormone hepcidin [22]. The mechanism by which HFE influences hepcidin expression is an area of current investigation and may offer insights into the phenotypic variability observed in persons with mutations in HFE [22]. A recent study suggests that less than 1% of subjects who are homozygous for the gene mutations will go on to develop the full-blown disease of hereditary hemochromatosis, historically termed "bronzed diabetes [24]." The study also suggests that homozygotes have no higher risk of mortality or of any clinically significant morbidity than normal control subjects [24]. The introduction of a commercially available genetic test for the C282Y and H63D mutations of HFE allows presymptomatic diagnosis, and adds precision to studies of the population genetics of HFE-related HH [25]. It is now recognized that a substantial proportion of C282Y homozygotes does not develop clinically significant iron overload, and modifier genes may be involved in this phenomenon [25]. Considering the duodenal crypt cell programming hypothesis, the recent discovery of HFE, the MHC-Class-I-like gene mutated in up to 90% of patients with hereditary haemochromatosis, and the gene encoding the Nramp2/divalent metal transporter-1 (DMT-1) implicated in ferrous iron transport holds promise for a greater understanding of human iron metabolism [26]. Caco-2 (small intestinal phenotype upon differentiation) and K562 (erythroleukaemic) HFE, in the presence of iron-saturated transferrin, co-localized with transferrin receptors in an early endosome compartment [26]. This interaction may be critical in small-intestinal crypt cells which express HFE, where it may function to modulate their intrinsic iron status thereby programming iron absorption by DMT-1 in the mature enterocyte [26]. Disruption of the HFE gene as a result of mutations associated with hereditary haemochromatosis may thus impair homeostatic mechanisms controlling iron absorption within the small-intestine epithelium by a direct interaction with transferrin receptors and by subsequent alteration of DMT-1 expression [26].

C. Clinical Manifestation

The clinical manifestation of herediatary hemochromatosis is very vary. The clinical manifestation usually correlates to the degree of iron overload. In addition, it also shows that hemochromatosis is a very complex disease and that the type of mutation can influence its clinical manifestation [17]. The disease is characterized by an inappropriately increased intestinal iron absorption leading to early abnormalities of iron parameters followed by iron deposition in different organs [27]. Excessive iron causes tissue damage and fibrosis, leading to organ failure [27]. Symptoms develop only after the marked accumulation of iron stores develop, which causes functional insufficiency of these organs [27-29]. The symptoms are often variable, nonspecific, and attributed to other diseases [28]. Common signs and symptoms seen in the primary care setting include fatigue, weakness, abdominal pain, palpitations, skin pigmentation changes, and arthropathy, but any symptom associated with organ damage may be reported [29-30]. Clinical complications appear late in life and include liver cirrhosis, diabetes, cardiomyopathy, hypogonadism, arthropathy, skin pigmentation and susceptibility to liver cancer [27]. Clinical symptoms develop only in homozygotes [27]. Heterozy-gotes may show abnormalities of iron parameters, but are not clinically affected, unless carriers of other conditions which modify iron metabolism, such as chronic liver diseases, beta-thalassemia trait or other haemolytic anemias [27]. The pathology in herediatary is common in the case with severe complications. Liver pathology is very specific. The pattern of fibrosis in the liver plus the abundant iron deposition in the liver and other organs separate this entity pathologically from other causes of liver failure [31]. Stainable iron is present in both hepatocytes and Kupffer cells is the hallmark of this disorder [32]. Hepatocellular carcinoma is usually considered to occur in cirrhotic livers and consequently measures for the early diagnosis of this complication are only recommended in this type of patient [33].

D. Laboratory Diagnosis

Diagnosis of iron overload can be suspected on the basis of clinical data, high transferrin saturation and/or serum ferritin values [34]. However, several hyperferritinemic conditions are not related to iron overload, but may imply severe disorders (inflammations, neoplasia) or a deregulation of ferritin synthesis (hereditary hyperferritinemia-cataract syndrome), and iron overload secondary to aceruloplasminemia, and the recently described dysmetabolic-associated liver iron overload syndrome, are characterized by low or normal transferrin saturation levels [34]. Early diagnosis requires a high index of suspicion and an awareness of the clinical features of herediatary hemochromatosis [28]. A high percentage of saturation of serum transferrin is the hallmark of the disorder, and serum ferritin concentration gives an approximate estimation of the size of iron stores. Serum iron, total iron-binding capacity, and ferritin levels are useful screening studies, but liver biopsy with quantitative chemical determination of iron concentration is essential to evaluate histopathological changes and to help distinguish hereditary hemochromatosis from secondary iron overload [28]. The cost-effectiveness and utility of large-scale screening for haemochromatosis have been questioned given that many individuals with the homozygous C282Y mutation do not have iron overload or end-organ damage [35]. A significant body of research over the last 10-20 years supports the hypothesis that screening for hereditary hemochromatosis may be cost-effective, given the low-cost, low-risk therapeutic options available for most homozygous individuals [36]. The factors that confound a straightforward test of this hypothesis include the fact that the disease is not fully penetrant and that, to achieve the anticipated life-year gains, therapy must be instituted before disease complications become irreversible [36]. However, the use of phenotypic tests, such as serum transferrin-iron saturation, for initial screening avoids the problem of the identification of non-expressing homozygotes [35]. Liver biopsy remains important in management to determine the presence or absence of cirrhosis, particularly amongst patients with serum ferritin levels greater than 1000 ng/mL or elevated liver enzymes [35]. Hepatic computed tomography, magnetic susceptometry, and nuclear magnetic resonance provide new noninvasive ways of determining hepatic iron content, but chemical estimation of iron in a percutaneous liver biopsy specimen remains the mainstay of diagnosis [37].

E. Treatment

Therapeutic phlebotomy remains the treatment and, if instituted early, will prevent many of the organ-specific complications [38]. Therapeutic phlebotomy at regular intervals is the mainstay of the treatment of this disease and the life expectancy of these patients is similar to that of the normal population if phlebotomy is started before the onset of irreversible organ damage [39-43]. Iron is best and quickly removed by weekly or twice-weekly phlebotomy of 500 ml, containing approximately 250 mg iron. One to 3 years of weekly phlebotomy may be required to reduce stores to normal. As a guide to long-term maintenance therapy, is recommended phlebotomy every 3 months and the serum ferritin level should be maintained by less than 50 ng/ml [42]. There is an interesting observation that blood concentrations of cadmium in subjects with herediatary on maintenance phlebotomy treatment, were significantly higher than in paired controls [40]. For most patients, phlebotomy is the preferred treatment option; iron chelation therapies are available for patients unable to tolerate phlebotomy [39]. Although phlebotomy therapy is effective in removing excess iron in hereditary hemochromatosis, chelation therapy is required in the treatment of many patients who have combined secondary and transfusional iron overload due to disorders in erythropoiesis [44].

Neonatal Hemochromatosis

Neonatal hemochromatosis is a rare gestational condition in which iron accumulates in the fetal tissues in a distribution like that seen in hereditary hemochromatosis [45-47]. Jaundice can be the most important manifestation of this disoder [48]. Extensive liver damage is the dominant clinical feature, with late fetal loss or early neonatal death [45]. When excess iron accumulation occurs in utero, as with neonatal hemochromatosis, the infant may be stillborn or present with advanced, overwhelming liver disease [49-50]. Liver failure can be seen and lead to death [49]. Neonatal hemochromatosis recurs within sibships at a rate higher than that predicted for autosomal-recessive inheritance, possibly suggesting the role of a maternal factor [45]. It has been suggested that neonatal hemochromatosis may represent an unusual manifestation of hereditary hemochromatosis, which is human leukocyte antigen

(HLA) linked [51]. However, Hardy et al found no evidence for major rearrangements or deletions in H- or L-apoferritin genes, in TfR genes, or within the HLA locus [51]. They also found no evidence for linkage of NH to HLA serotypes [51]. Hardy et al concluded that while neonatal hemochromatosis and herediatary were similar in their patterns of iron loading, they were not genetically related [51]. Silver et al suggested that, irrespective of the fetal liver disease being genetic or acquired, hepatic iron overload was directly involved in pathogenesis [52]. Knisely et al said that the abnormalities in cellular iron handling, undefined at present, that ere associated with the phenotype common to neontal hemochromatosis and adult idiopathic hemochromatosis did not appear primarily to involve the regulation by iron of rates of transferin receptor and ferritin synthesis [53].

Neonatal hemochromatosis should be suspected in the presence of cholestasis with liver failure of perinatal onset and with high blood level ferritin [54]. Abdominal nuclear magnetic resonance and/or liver biopsy can confirm neonatal hemochromatosis [54]. The pathology of neonatal hemochromatosis is characterized by severe fibrosis or cirrhosis and siderosis of the liver and other organs without affecting the mononuclear fagocytic system [55-57]. The ratio of iron concentration in the liver and spleen (1.5) allows to discard other causes of siderosis [55]. The defect features by severe prenatal iron storage in the liver and in a number of visceral organs similarly as in the hereditary adult type hemochromatosis [56]. Urinary cytology, serum iron concentration, iron-binding capacity, ferritin, and magnetic resonance imaging allow a diagnosis to be made before death [57]. Intrauterine diagnosis of perinatal hemochromatosis is difficult. Noninvasive detection of hepatic iron deposition is crucial [58]. By visual analysis, if the fetal liver is less intense than maternal or fetal fat signal for T2* gradient echo image, hemochromatosis should be suggested [58]. Earlier diagnosis may be required for optimal results [59].

Immunomodulation during pregnancy at risk appears to lessen the severity of disease [45]. Basically, hemochromatosis should be considered in the differential diagnosis of hydrops fetalis [60]. The recurrence risk is high, and immunomodulation with intravenous immunoglobulin treatment appears to alter the course of the disease with better infant survival [60]. IVIG, 1 g/kg bodyweight, weekly from the 18th week until the end of gestation in their subsequent pregnancy is recommended [61]. Treatment with high-dose IVIG during gestation appears to have modified recurrent neonatal haemochromatosis so that it is not lethal to the fetus or neonate [61]. For the affected infant, neonatal haemochromatosis can be a fatal disease with > 60% mortality [62]. Neonatal hemochromatosis carries a grim prognosis; however, successful orthotopic liver transplantation is curative [59]. Early treatment with antioxidant cocktail is beneficial and may be curative in those who present with milder phenotype [62]. However, the use of an antioxidant-chelation cocktail usually does not improve outcome in the patients [59]. Rodrigues et al reported that chelation-antioxidant treatment did not appear to modify the prognosis of neonatal hemochromatiosis [63]. Liver transplantation, with 50% long-term survival, remains the treatment of choice and should be promptly offered to those infants who do not improve with supportive medical treatment [63]. At this moment very early aggressive supportive treatment should appear to be the most useful approach to stabilize the patient hoping in spontaneous liver recovery, or, in turn, to permit transplantation before septic complications bring to clinical decline [64].

Hence, liver transplantation should always be considered at an early stage in non-responders and in children with more severe acute liver failure [62].

REFERENCES

[1] Oates PS, West AR. Heme in intestinal epithelial cell turnover, differentiation, detoxification, inflammation, carcinogenesis, absorption and motility. *World J Gastroenterol.* 2006 Jul 21;12(27):4281-95.

[2] Beaumont C. Molecular mechanisms of iron homeostasis. *Med Sci (Paris).* 2004 Jan;20(1):68-72.

[3] Fleming RE. Advances in understanding the molecular basis for the regulation of dietary iron absorption. *Curr Opin Gastroenterol.* 2005 Mar;21(2):201-6.

[4] Chung, Wessling-Resnick. Lessons learned from genetic and nutritional iron deficiencies. *Nutr Rev.* 2004 May;62(5):212-5.

[5] Tapiero H, Gate L, Tew KD. Iron: deficiencies and requirements. *Biomed Pharmacother.* 2001 Jul;55(6):324-32.

[6] Dunn LL, Rahmanto YS, Richardson DR. Iron uptake and metabolism in the new millennium. *Trends Cell Biol.* 2007 Feb;17(2):93-100.

[7] Ludwiczek S, Theurl I, Bahram S, Schumann K, Weiss G. Regulatory networks for the control of body iron homeostasis and their dysregulation in HFE mediated hemochromatosis. *J Cell Physiol.* 2005 Aug;204(2):489-99.

[8] Beaton MD, Adams PC. The myths and realities of hemochromatosis. *Can J Gastroenterol.* 2007 Feb;21(2):101-4.

[9] Beutler E. Hemochromatosis: genetics and pathophysiology. *Annu Rev Med.* 2006; 57:331-47.

[10] Ganz T. Hepcidin--a peptide hormone at the interface of innate immunity and iron metabolism. *Curr Top Microbiol Immunol.* 2006; 306:183-98.

[11] Verga Falzacappa MV, Muckenthaler MU. Hepcidin: iron-hormone and anti-microbial peptide. *Gene.* 2005 Dec 30;364:37-44.

[12] Galacteros F. Secondary iron overload. *Rev Prat.* 2000 May 1;50(9):983-7.

[13] Kushner JP, Porter JP, Olivieri NF. Secondary iron overload. *Hematology Am Soc Hematol Educ Program.* 2001; 47-61.

[14] Kontoghiorghes GJ, Pattichi K, Hadjigavriel M, Kolnagou A. Transfusional iron overload and chelation therapy with deferoxamine and deferiprone (L1). *Transfus Sci.* 2000 Dec;23(3):211-23.

[15] Franchini M. Recent acquisitions in the management of iron overload. *Ann Hematol.* 2005 Oct;84(10):640-5.

[16] Pietrangelo A. Hereditary hemochromatosis. *Annu Rev Nutr.* 2006; 26:251-70.

[17] Romanowski T, Sikorska K, Bielawski KP. Molecular basis of hereditary hemochromatosis. *Postepy Hig Med Dosw (Online).* 2006; 60:217-26.

[18] Franchini M. Hereditary iron overload: update on pathophysiology, diagnosis, and treatment. *Am J Hematol.* 2006 Mar;81(3):202-9.

[19] Beutler E. Hemochromatosis: genetics and pathophysiology. *Annu Rev Med.* 2006; 57:331-47.

[20] Zoller H, Cox TM. Hemochromatosis: genetic testing and clinical practice. *Clin Gastroenterol Hepatol.* 2005 Oct;3(10):945-58.

[21] Yen AW, Fancher TL, Bowlus CL. Revisiting hereditary hemochromatosis: current concepts and progress. *Am J Med.* 2006 May;119(5):391-9.

[22] Fleming RE, Britton RS, Waheed A, Sly WS, Bacon BR. Pathophysiology of hereditary hemochromatosis. *Semin Liver Dis.* 2005 Nov;25(4):411-9.

[23] Fleming RE, Britton RS, Waheed A, Sly WS, Bacon BR. Pathogenesis of hereditary hemochromatosis. *Clin Liver Dis.* 2004 Nov;8(4):755-73, vii.

[24] Neff LM. Current directions in hemochromatosis research: towards an understanding of the role of iron overload and the HFE gene mutations in the development of clinical disease. *Nutr Rev.* 2003 Jan;61(1):38-42.

[25] Britton RS, Fleming RE, Parkkila S, Waheed A, Sly WS, Bacon BR. Pathogenesis of hereditary hemochromatosis: genetics and beyond. *Semin Gastrointest Dis.* 2002 Apr;13(2):68-79.

[26] Griffiths WJ, Kelly AL, Smith SJ, Cox TM. Localization of iron transport and regulatory proteins in human cells. *QJM.* 2000 Sep;93(9):575-87.

[27] Camaschella C, Merlini R. Inherited hemochromatosis: from genetics to clinics. *Minerva Med.* 2005 Jun;96(3):207-22.

[28] Nichols GM, Bacon BR. Hereditary hemochromatosis: pathogenesis and clinical features of a common disease. *Am J Gastroenterol.* 1989 Aug;84(8):851-62.

[29] Stephenson D. Detecting hereditary hemochromatosis. *Nurse Pract.* 2000 Jul;25(7):64, 69, 73-6.

[30] Matthews AL, Grimes SJ, Wiesner GL, Acheson LS. Clinical consult: iron overload-hereditary hemochromatosis. *Prim Care.* 2004 Sep;31(3):767-70, xii-xiii.

[31] Ferrell L, Schmidt K, Sheffield V, Packman S. Neonatal hemochromatosis: genetic counseling based on retrospective pathologic diagnosis. *Am J Med Genet.* 1992 Nov 1;44(4):429-33.

[32] Lefkowitch JH. Hepatobiliary pathology. Curr Opin Gastroenterol. 2005May;21(3):260-9.

[33] Pellise M, Gonzalez-Abraldes J, Navasa M, Miquel R, Bruguera M. Hepatocellular carcinoma in a patient with hereditary hemochromatosis without cirrhosis. *Gastroenterol Hepatol.* 2001 Mar;24(3):132-4.

[34] Piperno A. Classification and diagnosis of iron overload. *Haematologica.* 1998 May;83(5):447-55.

[35] Whittington CA, Kowdley KV. Review article: haemochromatosis. *Aliment Pharmacol Ther.* 2002 Dec;16(12):1963-75.

[36] Buffone GJ, Beck JR. Cost-effectiveness analysis for evaluation of screening programs: hereditary hemochromatosis. *Clin Chem.* 1994 Aug;40(8):1631-6.

[37] Valberg LS, Ghent CN. Diagnosis and management of hereditary hemochromatosis. *Annu Rev Med.* 1985;36:27-37.

[38] Vautier G, Murray M, Olynyk JK. Hereditary haemochromatosis: detection and management. *Med J Aust.* 2001 Oct 15;175(8):418-21.

[39] Franchini M, Veneri D. Recent advances in hereditary hemochromatosis. *Ann Hematol.* 2005 Jun;84(6):347-52.

[40] Olynyk JK, Bacon BR. Hereditary hemochromatosis. Detecting and correcting iron overload. *Postgrad Med.* 1994 Oct;96(5):151-8, 161, 165.

[41] Akesson A, Stal P, Vahter M. Phlebotomy increases cadmium uptake in hemochromatosis. *Environ Health Perspect.* 2000 Apr;108(4):289-91.

[42] Dantas W. Hereditary hemochromatosis. *Rev Gastroenterol Peru.* 2001 Jan-Mar;21(1):42-55.

[43] Waalen J, Beutler E. Hereditary hemochromatosis: screening and management. *Curr Hematol Rep.* 2006 Mar;5(1):34-40.

[44] Britton RS, Leicester KL, Bacon BR. Iron toxicity and chelation therapy. *Int J Hematol.* 2002 Oct;76(3):219-28.

[45] Knisely AS, Mieli-Vergani G, Whitington PF. Neonatal hemochromatosis. *Gastroenterol Clin North Am.* 2003 Sep;32(3):877-89, vi-vii.

[46] Murray KF, Kowdley KV. Neonatal hemochromatosis. *Pediatrics.* 2001 Oct;108(4):960-4.

[47] Vohra P, Haller C, Emre S, Magid M, Holzman I, Ye MQ, Iofel E, Shneider BL. Neonatal hemochromatosis: the importance of early recognition of liver failure. *J Pediatr.* 2000 Apr;136(4):537-41.

[48] Burton BK. Inborn errors of metabolism in infancy: a guide to diagnosis. *Pediatrics.* 1998 Dec;102(6):E69.

[49] Whitington PF, Kelly S, Ekong UD. Neonatal hemochromatosis: fetal liver disease leading to liver failure in the fetus and newborn. *Pediatr Transplant.* 2005 Oct;9(5):640-5.

[50] Chase MC, Riedinger D. Neonatal hemochromatosis: a case report. *Neonatal Netw.* 1995 Oct;14(7):7-12.

[51] Hardy L, Hansen JL, Kushner JP, Knisely AS. Neonatal hemochromatosis. Genetic analysis of transferrin-receptor, H-apoferritin, and L-apoferritin loci and of the human leukocyte antigen class I region. *Am J Pathol.* 1990 Jul;137(1):149-53.

[52] Silver MM, Beverley DW, Valberg LS, Cutz E, Phillips MJ, Shaheed WA. Perinatal hemochromatosis. Clinical, morphologic, and quantitative iron studies. *Am J Pathol.* 1987 Sep;128(3):538-54.

[53] Knisely AS, Harford JB, Klausner RD, Taylor SR. Neonatal hemochromatosis. The regulation of transferrin-receptor and ferritin synthesis by iron in cultured fibroblastic-line cells. *Am J Pathol.* 1989 Feb;134(2):439-45.

[54] Liet JM, Urtin-Hostein C, Joubert M, Moussali F, David A, Nomballais F, Roze JC. Neonatal hemochromatosis. *Arch Pediatr.* 2000 Jan;7(1):40-4.

[55] Rodriguez Velasco A, Garcia GR, Tejeda Vega S, Sjordia Reyes GA, Ferman Cano F, Cantu Cuevas MA. Neonatal hemochromatosis. Report of 3 autopsy cases. *Rev Invest Clin.* 1999 Mar-Apr;51(2):81-7.

[56] Elleder M, Chlumska A, Hadravska S, Pilat D. Neonatal (perinatal) hemochromatosis. *Cesk Patol.* 2001 Nov;37(4):146-53.

[57] de Boissieu D, Badoual J. Perinatal hemochromatosis. *Pediatrie.* 1991; 46(2):141-5.

[58] Marti-Bonmati L, Baamonde A, Poyatos CR, Monteagudo E. Prenatal diagnosis of idiopathic neonatal hemochromatosis with MRI. *Abdom Imaging.* 1994 Jan-Feb;19(1):55-6.

[59] Sigurdsson L, Reyes J, Kocoshis SA, Hansen TW, Rosh J, Knisely AS. Neonatal hemochromatosis: outcomes of pharmacologic and surgical therapies. *J Pediatr Gastroenterol Nutr.* 1998 Jan;26(1):85-9.

[60] Venkat-Raman N, Venkata-Krishnan RV, Howarth ES. Successful pregnancy outcome following maternal intravenous immunoglobulin treatment in a woman with recurrent perinatal haemochromatosis. *Prenat Diagn.* 2006 Dec;26(13):1256-9.

[61] Whitington PF, Hibbard JU. High-dose immunoglobulin during pregnancy for recurrent neonatal haemochromatosis. *Lancet.* 2004 Nov 6-12;364(9446):1690-8.

[62] Flynn DM, Mohan N, McKiernan P, Beath S, Buckels J, Mayer D, Kelly DA. Progress in treatment and outcome for children with neonatal haemochromatosis. *Arch Dis Child Fetal Neonatal Ed.* 2003 Mar;88(2):F124-7.

[63] Rodrigues F, Kallas M, Nash R, Cheeseman P, D'Antiga L, Rela M, Heaton ND, Mieli-Vergani G. Neonatal hemochromatosis--medical treatment vs. transplantation: the king's experience. *Liver Transpl.* 2005 Nov;11(11):1417-24.

[64] Bellini C, Bonacci W, Serra G. Neonatal hemochromatosis: significance of early identification. *Acta Biomed Ateneo Parmense.* 2000; 71 Suppl 1:749-53. *J Pediatr Orthop.* 1984 Sep;4(5):630-2

INDEX

A

B

C

D

I

J

K

L

M

N

O

P

Q

R

S

T

U

V

W

X

Y

Z